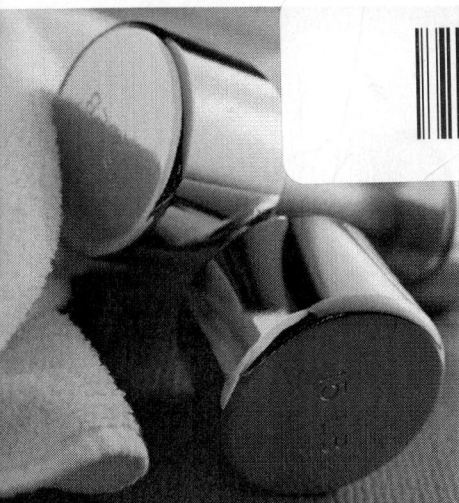

Entering the
Temple *of* Fitness

by Ron Emmons

Acknowledgements

I would like to thank Joanie Lawson my Marketing Specialist, Russell Adair for all the exercise photography and Ken Breivik, Nehemiah Communications for the introduction and production help.

For more Temple of Fitness information, visit www.TempleOfFitness.com

On the cover: Front row, l-r: Clarence Major, David Thomas.
Back row, l-r: Stephanie Bess, Ron Emmons and Louise Smith.

Entering the Temple of Fitness
by Ron Emmons
© Copyright 2006 Ron Emmons

Printed in the U.S.A. by Instantpublisher.com

ISBN 1-59196-655-8

Contents

Chapter		Page
1	Introduction	5
2	Dumbbells	9
3	The Basics	15
4	Upper Body	23
5	Lower Body	41
6	Abdominals	55
7	Eating Smart	57
8	The Temple of Fitness Workout for Men and Women	71
	About the Author	77

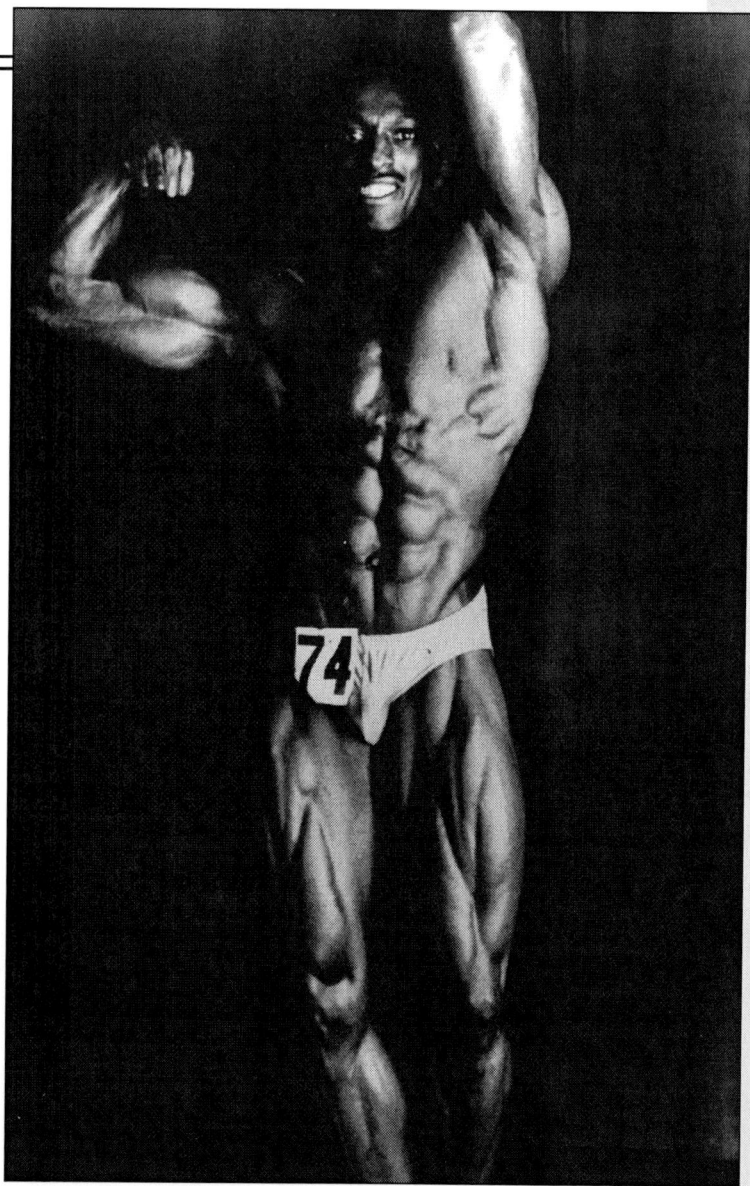

CHAPTER 1

Introduction

By Kenneth Breivik

L ike many people, a few years ago I set another new year's resolution to lose weight. I had tried various diets, exercise techniques and spent money on a variety of exercise equipment, only to lose a few pounds that I would eventually gain back. My wife had met Ron Emmons and recommended that I work out with him and see if it would make a difference. In January 2005 I met Ron for the first time. What impressed me about Ron was the great physical shape he was in and I was surprised to find that he was a few years older then me. Ron, who is a former professional body builder, has been asked over the years to train both recruits who are trying to meet their physical training (PT) requirements for the military and a variety of professional athletes.

He began by altering my diet and asking me to do the exercises outlined in "Entering the Temple of Fitness." Within one year I had lost almost 50 pounds and gone from a 46 waist to a 38. I feel like I am in better condition in my 40's then I was in my 30's. Ron and I got into a discussion about the links between physical and spiritual health, which he asked me to share as an introduction to this book.

There are three key concepts in the Bible that link physical training with spiritual health.

Key Concept: While Spiritual Fitness is more important, the Bible affirms the positive aspects of physical training.

In 1 Timothy 4:8 (NIV) Paul says, *"For physical training is of some value, but godliness has value for all things holding promise for both the present life and the life to come."* In this letter Paul is encouraging Timothy about the significance of his own spiritual training and its importance. It is interesting that Paul does not say that physical training does not have value. In fact Paul believes it has value during our life. The advantage of spiritual training is that we get the benefits both here on earth and in heaven.

While having our heart right with God and caring for other people give both an immediate benefit and an eternal benefit, which is more important? Paul understood that a person who is physically fit would have better health, a better quality of life and be in better physical shape to do whatever work God has given them to do. These benefits are all of tremendous help in our day-to-day lives. While I do remember being sore the first few times that I worked out using the methods in this book, overall I find that I get less tired and have more energy now that I am not carrying all the extra weight.

Key Concept: Paul and the other writers of the Bible use training and sports as a frequent example of spiritual life.

In 1 Corinthians 9:24-27, Paul writes, *"Do you know that in a race all the runners run, but only one gets the prize? Run in such a way as to get the prize. Everyone who competes in the games goes into strict training. They do it to get a crown that will not last; but we do it to get a crown that will last forever. Therefore I do not run like a man running aimlessly. I do not fight like a man beating the air. No, I beat my body and make it my slave so that after I have preached to others, I myself will not be disqualified for the prize."*

Many of the examples that are used in the Bible compare spiritual things with things that we experience everyday. For example, marriage is used to symbolize Christ's relationship to the church. The story of the talents uses business concepts as a parallel to both stewardship and putting our own "talents" to use. Through physical training we can see parallels to being in good "spiritual shape". A person, who says they love God, but does not pray, attend church, serve others or read the Bible is in bad spiritual shape. Just like in the physical realm, without proper diet, cardio and weight training a person cannot be in good physical shape.

I have also learned a number of life lessons from physical training. There is never an immediate "pay out" from exercise. The rewards are seen over time. Likewise, when we make changes in our spiritual habits, the rewards may be evident many months or even years later. That is why some people who do not learn this lesson stop their physical or spiritual training after only a short period of time. They want the payoff, but are not willing to work for their dreams.

Key Concept: Our bodies are a place for the Spirit of God to dwell and as such we should do good things to our body and not bad.

We have all heard the phrase, "your body is a temple", but have you ever thought about what it means so that it is a place for God to dwell? The thought behind this phrase comes from 1 Corinthians 6:19-20 which says, *"Do you not know that your body is a temple of the Holy Spirit, who is in you, whom you have received from God? You are not your own; you were bought at a price. Therefore honor God with your body."*

God cares both how you live your life and how you treat your body. Poor fitness and overeating are harmful to us and a bad witness to others. It is unfortunate that in our generation many people judge us by our outward appearance more than our inward beauty. However, we should not be discouraged by this, but encouraged to take seriously how we treat our bodies.

As you read, "Entering the Temple of Fitness" and learn about the proper way to exercise and the importance of and what a proper diet is, do not just focus on the goal of being physically fit, but on the goals of being fit in all areas of your life. As you achieve fitness in one area it is often an aid to achieving fitness in other areas of your life. I have a great respect for Ron Emmons and the knowledge and passion he has for physical fitness. In reading this book you will get an opportunity to benefit from his knowledge. He can be as real a help to you as he has been to me. Now it is time to enter the Temple of Fitness…

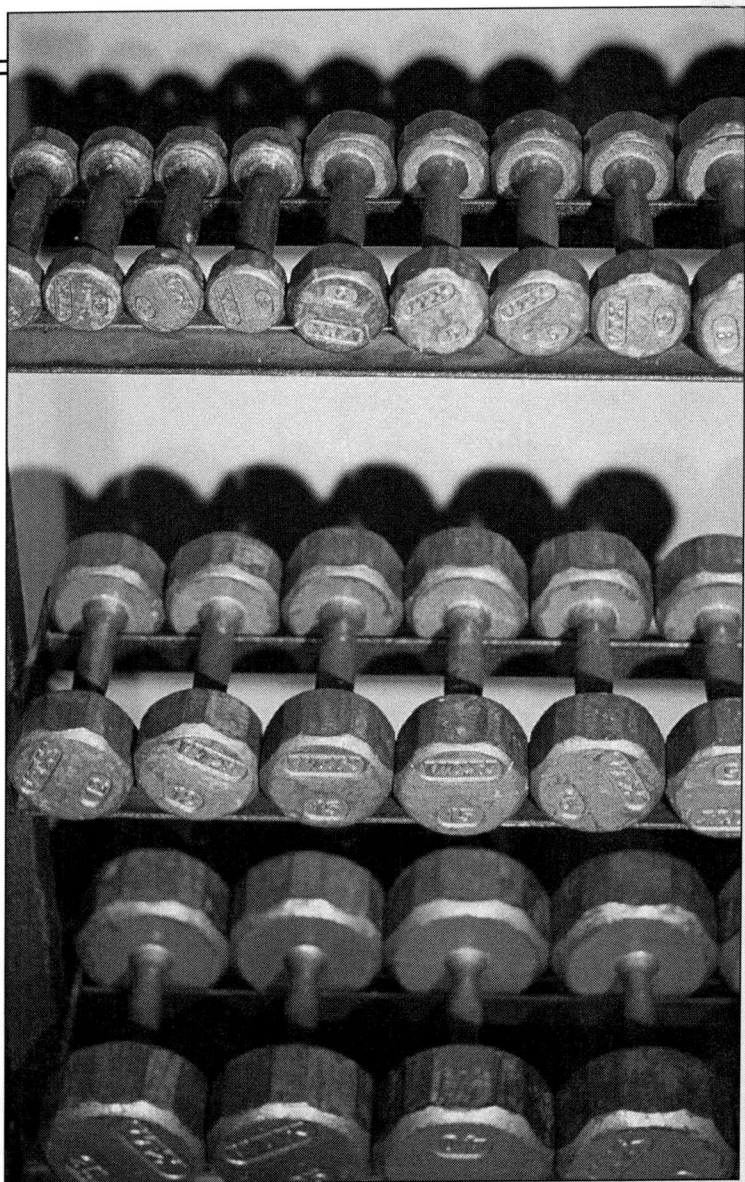

CHAPTER 2

Dumbbells

The Best, Easiest and Safest Way to Build Strength

I get the question all the time:

What is the best machine to help get in shape?

My answer is always the same:

"Dumbbells."

Dumbbells are by far and away the best, easiest, safest, cheapest, most convenient way to build strength. I know this flies in the face of infomercials selling hope (or is it hype?) in a box for three easy installment payments. I also know it runs counter to high-tech health clubs that market themselves by suggesting that if you hang with them and do their thing, you'll be dating models in no time. But the truth is, if you go to anyone who is serious about getting fit and strong— and staying fit and strong—you won't see a basement full of machines and mail-order belly busters.

What you'll see is dumbbells.

Here's why.

Dumbbells give you a greater range of motion. They don't limit your movements. For example, think about doing bench presses. You're on your back, you lift the bar, and then you ease it down. How far down? Until your chest gets in the way. With dumbbells, though, since you have one in each hand, you can bring the weights lower—as far past your chest line as possible—with each repetition. Those extra few inches are the key to faster muscle growth.

Machines restrict you in their own way, too. You push up and down, side to side, and back and forth. There's no way to adjust your lift or angle the weights in a certain direction—both of which not only strengthen the muscles, but also reduce stress on your joints. The machine determines what you do and how you do it, and there's typically only one way— because that's the way the equipment was designed.

With machines and barbells, the workout is basically over once you've exercised the muscle to exhaustion. But with dumbbells, some additional negative resistance training can be done. When you've maxed out on your reps, for example, use one arm to help the other do a few more, slowly, paying special attention to lowering the weight.

Dumbbells make you stronger faster.
Among bodybuilders, it's pretty much accepted that you can get quicker results from lowering the weight than you do from actually lifting it. Some machines are actually designed to minimize this motion, called "resistance," to make it easier on the user. All that does is reduce the positive effects of the workout.

With machines and barbells, the workout is basically over once you've exercised the muscle to exhaustion. But with dumbbells, some additional negative resistance training can be done. When you've maxed out on your reps, for example, use one arm to help the other do a few more, slowly, paying special attention to lowering the weight. The last two or three reps can increase the benefits—and the pay off—big time.

Dumbbells fit anyone's physical type.
Let's face it: When fitness machines are mass-produced, they are made to fit a "typical" or "average" body type. The problem is that not everyone fits so neatly into those categories. That raises the possibility that someone who isn't the ideal fit runs a risk of injury. Dumbbells, on the other hand, are much more democratic. They don't care who you are or what you look like. They don't care if you're young or old, male or female. They don't make any assumptions about you. They work for everyone.

Dumbbells better reflect actual body movements. Often, machines aren't conformed to fit the body, so when you use them you end up in a position that isn't even close to natural. This can put unhealthy stress on the muscle groups you're supposed to be strengthening and toning. Dumbbells let you work your muscles from different angles. This permits a workout that can actually imitate the motions you put your body through every day, as well as reduce joint stress.

Dumbbells make you think. Forget their name for a second. Dumbbells are no dummies. They force you to handle the weight, to concentrate and think about it. That puts more stress on the targeted muscle group, which in turn shapes them and tones them more effectively. Machines pretty much do the thinking for you. The weights are already balanced. All you do is climb in, sit down, and push and pull. That's it. Dumbbells don't allow an "auto-pilot" mentality.

Dumbbells correct muscle imbalance. For whatever reason, most people are stronger on one side of the body than the other. When barbells and machines are used, the strong side often makes up for the weak side, causing a further strength imbalance. Dumbbells don't care which side is stronger. They don't let you trick your left arm into thinking it's strong just because the right arm is covering for it. When you're using dumbbells, you typically have a weight gripped in each hand; and you have to use it.

Dumbbells are versatile. With a good dumbbell workout, you can strengthen just about every muscle in your body. That means you won't have to buy a machine for the back; and another one for the biceps; and another one for the chest; and another one for the shoulders' and another one for the triceps; and another one for...

Dumbbells are cheap. A good single machine—a machine that works just one muscle group—costs more than $1,000. A set of dumbbells ranging from 1 to 10 pounds will run you less than $35.00; and you can work all the muscle groups. What a deal!

Dumbbells take up less space. There's a reason gyms are the size of city blocks. They need all that room for all the individual machines that only work one muscle group. Try putting one of those machines into a footlocker, or tossing it in the back of your car. Dumbbells can be stowed anywhere, and they won't be in the way.

Dumbbells are safer. You don't need a spotter. The body is not being forced to do something it's not shaped for. Your joints are not being over stressed. There's no chance a 20-pound bar and 100 pounds of iron are going to come crashing down on your chest.

Dumbbells can help prevent injury. Most machines work one specific muscle group. But in doing so, they ignore the ligaments, tendons and smaller muscles that keep your joints in shape. Dumbbells work those "forgotten areas" in addition to building strength in the larger muscle groups.

Don't get me wrong here. I'm not saying that barbells and machines are bad. The truth is any exercise activity-provided you do it right-is going to help. The question isn't, "What works?" The question is, "What works best?"

And as far as I am concerned, the answer is dumbbells. Hands down.

RON'S RULES TO WORK OUT BY

- Be mentally prepared.

- Wear the proper attire, especially loose-fitting clothes. Dress for comfort, not style.

- Use safety with weights. Lift smart.

- Find the weight appropriate for your exercise.

- Don't try to do too much too fast.

- Keep the proper form when exercising. Poor technique leads to injuries.

- Use the proper breathing technique. Inhale as you lower the weight, exhale as you lift it. Don't hold your breath.

- Don't over-extend your body and muscles. Listen to what you're body is telling you. When it's tired, pay attention.

- Don't over train. There is a point when too much weight work becomes counter-productive.

- Always use belts with squats or bent-over movements.

- Don't lock your knees and elbows. It puts too much stress on your bones.

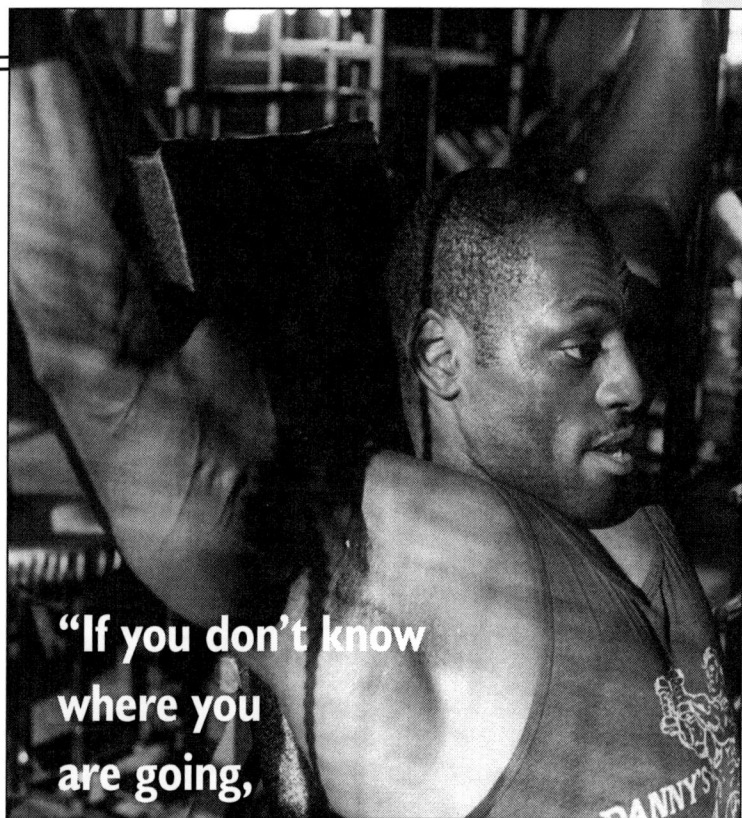

"If you don't know where you are going, you'll end up somewhere else."

– Ron Emmons

CHAPTER 3

The Basics

There's a saying in the military that goes something like this: The more you sweat in training, the less you bleed in war.

The thought behind that is simple. Anyone who is properly prepared to undertake a task will do it better, safer, smarter and more productively when the time comes to execute the task.

Strength training is the same. If you jump into it without learning the right techniques, you're asking to get hurt. If you don't know the right way to breathe, you could pass out. If you don't listen to your body—and it can tell you a lot—you may be ignoring signs that can prevent serious injury.

> "It is God who arms me with strength and makes my way perfect."
>
> – 2 Samuel 22:33 (NIV)

So, the purpose of this chapter is pretty basic: getting started on the right foot, and making sure you know where you're going. Because the fact is, if you don't know where you're going, you'll end up somewhere else; and, when we're talking about doing what's right and best for your body, that's the last place you want to be.

Some basic definitions

Some terms will be used over and over in this book, so I want to make sure we're all on the same page and there's no room for misunderstanding or misinterpretation.

> One of the easiest ways to really injure yourself in training is to try to lift too much weight, too fast, too early in the process.

Chair or Bench. Chairs come in all kinds of styles and prices. Whatever kind you prefer (the most expensive is not necessarily the best.), make sure you use one that is sturdy enough to hold your weight and doesn't wobble beneath you. In addition to flattening out, the back of the bench should be adjustable to both a 45-degree and a 90-degree angle.

Dumbbells. These are short-handled barbells. They range in weight from 1 pound to as much as 180 pounds, and come in all kinds of shapes and styles: hexagonal (to keep from rolling around), round (if rolling around doesn't bother you), plastic, cast iron, adjustable (with sleeves and clamps that allow you to adjust the amount of weight rather than having a different dumbbell for every weight class). For training purposes, you should get a pair of dumbbells for each of the following weights: 1, 2, 3, 4, 5 and 8 lbs.

Form. This refers to the biomechanics of a weight-training movement. In other words, it's how you do the exercise. Perfect form involves using only the muscles that are specific to a given exercise while moving the weights over the fullest possible range of motion.

Repetition or Rep. This is the single full range of movement in an exercise. For example, if you were doing a shoulder press, raising the dumbbells and then lowering them back to the starting position would make up one rep.

Routine. The total number of exercises, sets and reps used during a single training session. In the Temple of Fitness routine, you do 21 exercises, from 1 to 3 sets each and 12 to 15 reps per set.

Set. Refers to the specific number of reps performed during a single unit of a single exercise.

What to wear

The object of weight training isn't to get noticed. The object is to get fit. Forget about making a fashion statement and stick to the basics: shorts, sweats, T-shirt or tank top, leg tights, warm-up suits, etc. I prefer to wear shoes that are designed primarily for running because they offer the best arch support. There are also a lot of cross-trainers on the market that work just as well. The key to a good shoe is comfort. If it feels good, wear it.

Warming up

If you've been working out your entire life or are picking up a dumbbell for the first time, you still need to warm up. The 5 to 8 minutes you spend prepping for your routine are just as important as the 45 minutes or so you'll spend actually doing the exercises. By taking the time to warm up your muscles, they will become more flexible and less likely to get injured. The best, easiest warm-up exercises are light calisthenics (jumping jacks, toe touches or running in place), an easy jog or fast walk, a few minutes on a stationary bike or some simple stretching.

> If you've been working out your entire life or are picking up a dumbbell for the first time, you still need to warm up.

How much weight? How many reps? How often?

One of the easiest ways to really injure yourself in training is to try to lift too much weight, too fast, too early in the process. While that's true for just about everyone, it is especially the case if you're a beginner, aren't used to dumbbell workouts or haven't been exercising for an extended period of time. Given that a key objective of dumbbell training is to avoid injury (How can you get your body in peak shape if you're too hurt to work out?), I'd recommend these weight levels as starting points for the Temple of Fitness routine:

Muscle Group	Exercise	Weight (Men)	Weight (Women)
Chest	Press	5 pounds	1 pound
Chest	Fly	5 pounds	1 pound
Shoulders	Press	5 pounds	1 pound
Shoulders	Side Laterals	3 pounds	1 pound
Shoulders	Front Laterals	3 pounds	1 pound
Back	Bent-Over Row (Forward grip)	8 pounds	3 pounds
Back	Bent-Over Row (Reverse grip)	8 pounds	3 pounds
Back	One Arm Row	8 pounds	5 pounds
Biceps	Seated Curl	8 pounds	5 pounds
Triceps	Double Arm Overhead Extensions	5 pounds	3 pounds
Triceps	Double Arm Kickback	5 pounds	3 pounds
Legs	Squats	8 pounds	5 pounds
Legs	Angle Squats	8 pounds	5 pounds
Legs	Hack Squats	8 pounds	5 pounds
Legs	Stiff Leg Dead Lifts	8 pounds	5 pounds
Legs	Calf Raises	8 pounds	5 pounds

Start Smart. When you're first starting out, do one set of 15 reps per exercise. Sure, you may want to do more than 15, but guess what? More are not going to make you any stronger or improve your endurance. So why waste the time and effort?

Also, don't even consider doing fewer reps with heavier weights. For some reason, people believe that will bulk them up. It won't. About the only thing it does is increase the potential for injury—especially pulled muscles.

Adding Weight. Obviously, it's going to become easier and easier to lift the weights as you work out more. That's good. It shows you're getting stronger. But don't let all this newfound strength go to your head and trick you into thinking you can suddenly jump from 1.5 pounds to 30 pounds just because you feel like Superman or Superwoman. Rather, you always adjust up a single weight level: 2 pounds to 3; 4 to 5; 5 to 6; etc.

How do you know when it's time to make the leap? Consider this: as long as the last three reps in a set are hard to finish, and you still feel the muscles burning at that point in the exercise, you don't need to increase your weights. But if you're coasting through a set and the last three are only slightly tougher than the first three, go for it.

One other thing about weights. The amount of weight you can lift is going to vary from day to day. Some days, you're just not going to hit the levels you usually hit. There could be a lot of reasons for this from a lack of sleep to a nutritional imbalance to the fact that it's been a tough day and you're just exhausted. Don't think of that as some kind of setback, because it's not. It just means the body is telling you to chill out.

And don't make the mistake of ignoring the message by busting your hump to get to that previous level. If you're tired but try to press on, you're asking for all kinds of injuries, from strained and pulled muscles to undue stress on your bones and joints. It's okay to have an off day every once in a while. Don't sweat it.

Resting Between Sets. I'm not real big on saying you should take an exact amount of time between sets. Everyone's body is different, and we all respond differently to the stress of exercise, so it just seems a little pointless to force different kinds of people into a hard-and-fast formula.

I suggest that after finishing a set, you rest until your breathing returns to normal, and then continue. For some people, that may be 30 seconds; for others, 45 seconds or even a minute. Like I said before—and I'll say it a lot in this book—the point is to pay attention to what you're body is telling you. When your heart rate slows down after a tough set, that's the signal it's the right time to go on.

Multiple Sets. As your strength increases and a single routine isn't quite so tough to get through, you might want to move up to multiple sets—two or three per exercise. Provided you maintain the proper form and don't try to overdo it, multiple or super-sets can deliver a lot of benefits and improve your performance. It will take a little more time, that's true. But the payback can be awesome.

When you move to multiple sets, there is the chance you may not be able to lift the same weights through out each set. That's natural, and nothing to worry about. You're just putting each muscle group to maximum stress, which is a good thing. However, when you're on that second or third set and you feel like you just can't do any more—stop. Don't force your muscles to do things they can't do. If you hit the wall midway through a set, simply drop down to the next weight level and finish up. You are still be working the muscles to the max, but you'll be doing it smart and avoiding the kinds of injuries that come with over use.

Frequency. Finally, let's talk about how often workouts should be. One of the best things about the Temple of Fitness routine is its efficiency. It doesn't take a lot of time—30 or 45 minutes tops for a single set. Since most muscle groups except the abs need 48 hours of rest between workouts (abs can be worked every day if you want), a three-day-a-week regimen is ideal. While your schedule will determine when you train, a Monday-Wednesday-Friday program is usually the best bet.

Form

In later chapters, I explain the proper form for each exercise in the Temple of Fitness routine. But there is one point that I can't stress too much, and you will see it repeatedly throughout this book:

Go slow.

It's not just a matter of being careful, concentrating and making sure the exercise is done the right way. The slower you go, the more the muscle is worked. That's particularly the case in the resistance phase of the repetition, which is a high-strength motion.

Some people suggest that you should spend two seconds lifting the weight and two seconds lowering it. Others say taking four seconds to bring it down maximizes the benefit of the resistance motion. Again, I'm not a fan of easy formulas. Just remember to take it slow. Keep every movement even, smooth and deliberate whether you're raising the dumbbell or lowering it.

There is one other bit of advice that you'll see popping in and out of the instruction. **Never lock your knees or elbows in any of the exercises.** It takes the stress off the muscle and puts it right on the bones. So you're not only cutting the muscles some slack— which defeats the whole purpose of working out—but you're also putting a ton of stress on your joints. And that's bad news.

Breathing

There is a tendency during a workout to hold your breath when lifting weights. I don't know why. But for some reason, people tend to suck in a lung full of air and then just keep it there.

Let me be blunt. **Holding your breath during a routine can be a ticket to blacking out.**

Lifting weights increases your blood pressure. Holding your breath increases it even more. Not only that, but it cuts off the oxygen supply to your brain which means you're begging for a fainting spell.

Breathing is as important a part of the Temple of Fitness routine as the exercises themselves. Like everything else, there's a right way to and a wrong way to breathe.

The right way is to inhale as you lower the weight, exhale as you lift it. With squats, inhale as you lower the body and exhale as you return to position, it's simple and helps your body get in a kind of aerobic rhythm that will help you reach and maintain peak performance.

Belts

There are some people who will tell you that weight belts are actually counterproductive in the workout because the belt—not the muscles— stabilizes the body. I am not one of those people.

Belts provide support and protection. Even at minimum exertion, both men and women should wear a belt during leg training to prevent back injury and keep the abdominal muscles from protruding. This is not optional. Not doing so presents a risk that's as real as it gets. In fact, you should wear a belt not only for lower-body workouts, but also for every back exercise except the one-arm row. As for wearing one during the other parts of the Temple of Fitness routine, it's your call. But since I'm a big believer in injury avoidance, I don't think you can ever be too careful.

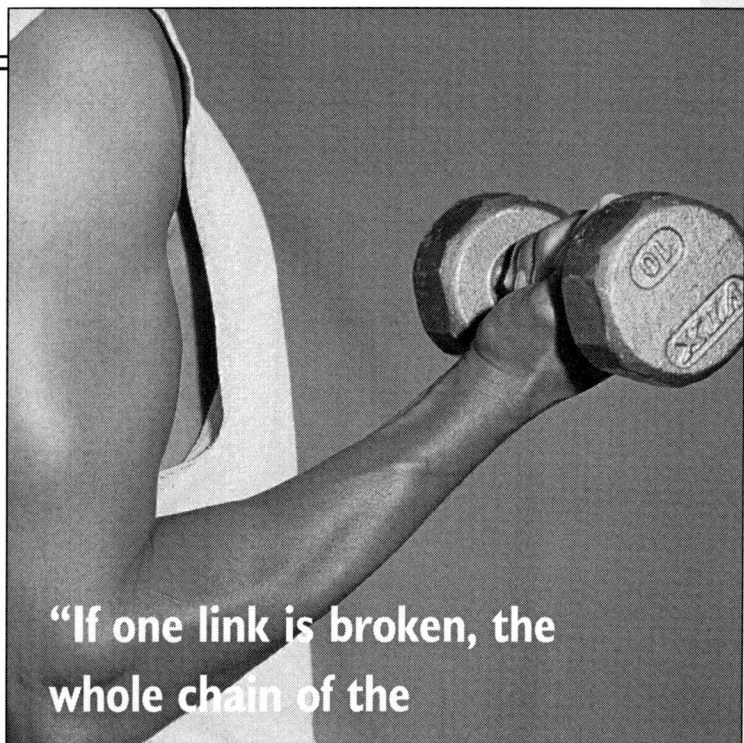

"If one link is broken, the whole chain of the upper body strength will suffer."

– Ron Emmons

CHAPTER 4

Upper body

Face the facts: If you want to do a lot of pushups, you have to get your upper body in shape. I'm not just talking about your arms; or your shoulders; or your chest; or your back.

I'm talking about the total package. All of it.

Think about the basic mechanics of a pushup. You're stretched out, palms on the floor, and up on your toes. Gradually, you lift your body by straightening out your arms and pushing away from the floor. Just before your elbows lock, you slowly lower yourself back down. Throughout the entire exercise, you keep yourself rigid and straight as a ruler.

Easy, right? Your arms are doing all the heavy lifting, nothing to it.

Not exactly.

Consider the range of motion a single pushup requires. First, you bring your body up and then you drop it down. That's good arm work, and you can thank your biceps and triceps for making it happen. What permits your arms to do these things and distributes the burden throughout the upper body as opposed to concentrating it on just one overworked muscle group? Your shoulders. And what's giving your shoulders the support they need to get you through a pushup without any collateral damage? Your chest and back.

> "He has performed mighty deeds with his arms, he has scattered those who are proud in their inmost thought."
> – Luke 1:51 (NIV)

It's like the chain of command. In the military or business world, if there's a breakdown at any point in the process, then the whole process suffers. The same principle applies to your upper body. Arm action is linked to shoulder strength, and shoulder strength is linked to chest and upper-back strength. If any of these links is weak, then the whole chain of strength will suffer. The primary function of any upper-body workout is to make sure that doesn't happen and to train each muscle group to perform its part safely, effectively and efficiently.

Get up in arms

Arms are basically made up of two muscle groups: biceps and triceps. The biceps are located on the front of your upper arms, stretching from the elbows to the shoulders. Their primary function is to bend the arm. So if you're tugging or jerking at something, lowering yourself on a pushup or even curling your arm to drink a cup of coffee, the biceps are doing the work.

These muscles are like the crown jewels of weight work. Often, when people start working out, their goal is to get biceps that look like cantaloupes when they flex. That's okay, but remember, they're just one part of the upper body package. Impressive biceps may be nice, and get you a lot of attention in the gym but they're not going to do you a lot of good if your triceps, shoulders, chest and back aren't strong enough to do their part of the heavy lifting.

A real danger with concentrating solely on the biceps is that you neglect your triceps, which are located on the underside of the arm. For all the attention people put on the biceps, it's the triceps that make up about 60 percent of the arm muscles. They allow you to straighten the arm out. When a referee signals a touchdown, he's using the triceps. After your biceps let you cock your arm to throw a baseball, the triceps let you follow through. Once you've dropped down into a pushup position, it's the triceps that let you come back up.

They may not look as cool as biceps, and my guess is you're not going to hear many people say, "Wow, awesome triceps!" But the fact remains, you can't ignore them. If you do, you'll risk a strength imbalance in your upper arms that can lead to muscle tears. And if that happens, you're going to have a tough time doing so much as one pushup.

Shouldering the burden of motion

Your shoulders are like command central for a whole range of arm movements. Called the deltoid muscles, they stretch from the top of the upper arm down to about the middle. Because of their structure—the joint is like a ball and socket, with the ball of the arm fitting into the socket of the shoulder—they make it easy to move your arms in just about any direction.

Strong shoulders do more than just make arm motions easier. They also make sure that your back and chest don't do all the work when you're exercising. By "shouldering the burden" of weight work, your delts can help prevent tears in other muscle groups.

It is this same ball-and-joint structure that lets you swing your arms in every direction that is also a magnet for injuries. Look at the sports pages during the baseball season, and it's likely you'll read about a pitcher tearing his rotator cuff—the muscles and tendons that that keep your arm in the socket. Trust me, you don't have to throw hundred-mile-an-hour fastballs for this to happen to you. It can happen to anyone—especially if your workout form is slack or you try to hot-dog it by lifting too much weight before your body is ready. Moreover, since the deltoids cover your rotator cuff, it makes a lot of sense to keep them fit and strong.

A pec on the chest

If you go into just about any gym in the country and listen to a couple of bodybuilders talking to each other, I guarantee that at some point one will ask the other: How much can you bench?

They're not talking about using their shoulders or quads or triceps. They're talking about a chest press, which is pretty much the King of the World when it comes to popularity.

The chest muscles—notably the pectorals—are front and center when it comes to a full range of important movements such as lifting, pushing and hugging. On top of that, since the chest and shoulder muscles are connected, strong pecs can prevent a lot of the nagging—and potentially serious—injuries to your deltoids and rotator cuffs.

But for all of their benefits, don't fall too madly in love with chest exercise. Remember the pushup, and how total upper body conditioning is a function of arm, shoulder, back and chest strength. If you spend too much time on one muscle group and not enough on the others, you're risking serious injury. But regardless of whether it leads to an injury or compounds a strength imbalance, you'll never achieve the your peak level of performance.

Back to basic strength

For strength purposes, when I talk about the back I'm referring to the muscles in your upper back—specifically the latissimus dorsi. The lats start at your armpits and extend to the middle of your lower back, and you use them to do things like row a boat or carry your gear.

There are a couple of things you should never forget when you're working out the lats. The first is to remember that, as I said above, they focus on the upper back. Injuries to the lower back—which are where a lot of nagging problems occur, especially in men—can be prevented by stretching during the warm-up. If you do have back problems, be careful. Even the slightest deviation from perfect form can make a good back go bad and a bad back even worse.

Second, remember that it's the upper back muscles you are working. During the routine, there might be a tendency to let your arms and shoulders do too much work just because you're lifting dumbbells. Don't let it happen. Concentrate on your back muscles with every movement in order to benefit the most from each exercise.

The exercises

When doing an upper-body workout, always perform the exercises in the following order: chest, shoulders, back, biceps and triceps. If you mix up the sequence, the smaller muscles—mostly the biceps and triceps—will suck out the energy you need to work the larger muscle groups, which means you are going to burn out more quickly.

Fatigue doesn't simply exhaust your muscles. It can harm them, too, especially if you keep pushing yourself even when the body has other ideas. Starting your routine with the upper body workout—and then doing each of the exercises in the right order—will not only help you maximize the strength benefits but also minimize the risk of injury that comes from asking your muscles to do things they're not ready to do.

Throughout all exercise regimens, it's important to keep a smooth, easy rhythm. Don't go too fast, and don't get into the habit of jerking the dumbbells into position when you're lifting. That's bad form, and it's also dangerous. Always go slow, pay attention to your form, breathe right and concentrate on the muscle group you're working.

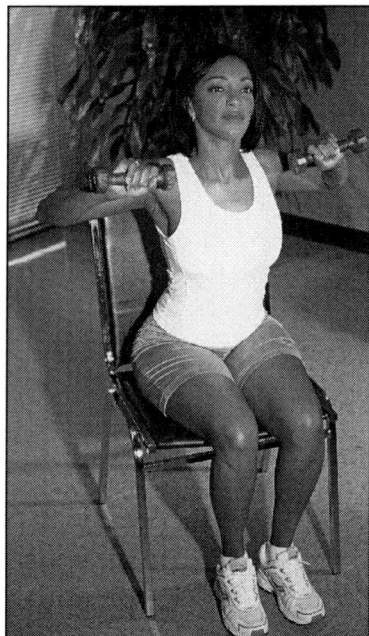

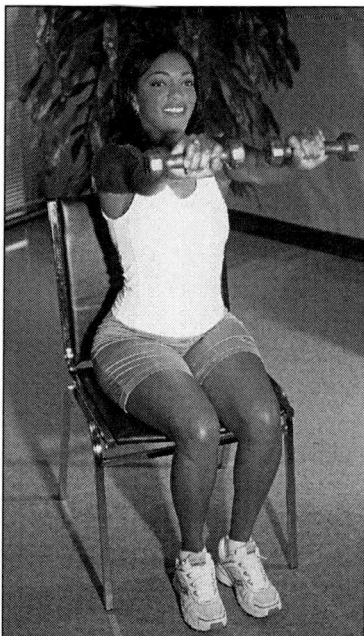

Dumbbell chest press

Sit upright in a chair with your legs slightly apart and feet firmly on the ground. Start by holding the dumbbells, palms facing down and close to your armpits. As the weights are pressed outward, begin to bring them closer together, slowly and evenly, as you extend your arms.

Stop when the inside ends of the weights are about an inch or an inch and a half apart and your arms are fully extended. Return to the starting position, following the same path you used on the outward press, to ensure a full range of motion.

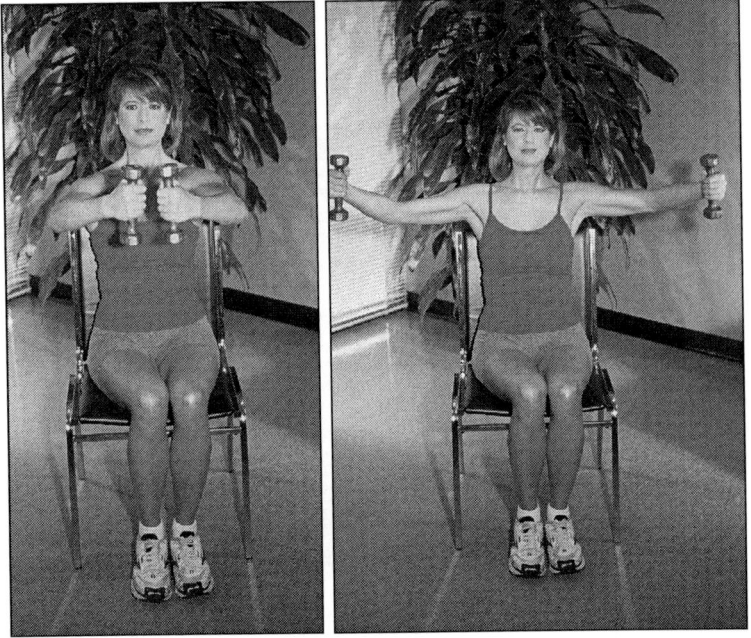

Seated upright flye (chest)

Sitting upright in a chair, hold the dumbbells straight out in front of your body, palms facing each other, wrists slightly turned in towards each other. Don't lock your elbows. Keeping your arms parallel to the floor, move the dumbbells outward away from each other in a semicircular motion until they are at minimum level with your chest.

Once maximum rotation has been reached, bring the dumbbells back up in the same semicircular motion—imagine you're hugging a tree—until they've returned to the starting position.

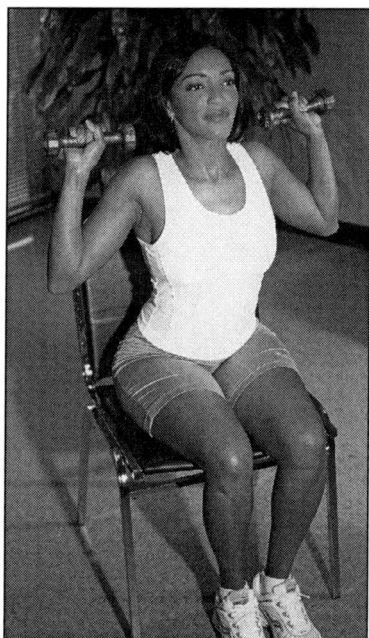

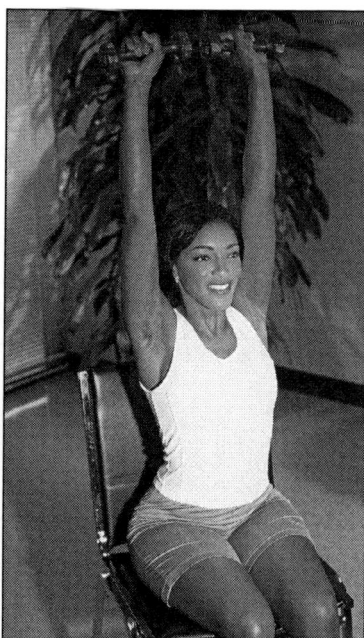

Dumbbell shoulder press (shoulders)

Sit upright in the chair with your back straight, legs comfortably apart and feet firmly on the ground. Hold your upper arms straight out, bent at the forearms so that the dumbbells are about even with your ears. Grip them with your palms facing out. Slowly lift the weights up and toward each other stopping when the ends are an inch or an inch and a half apart. Just as slowly, return the dumbbells to the starting position at ear-level. Keep your back straight and your body still throughout. Don't lock your elbows at any point in the movement.

Dumbbell side laterals (shoulders

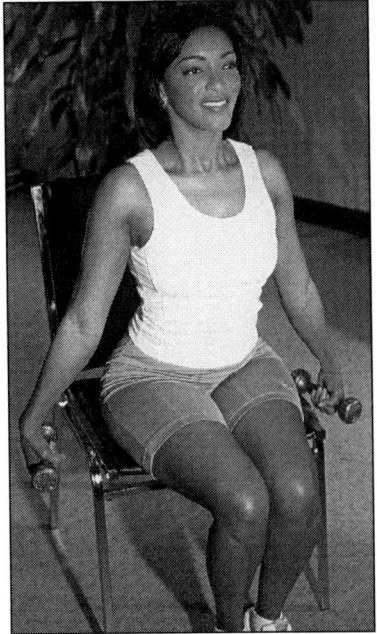

Sit upright in the chair, as in the previous exercise. Let your arms extend fully to your side, holding the dumbbells with your palms facing down, wrists curled down slightly. Raise your arms slowly — away from your body, straight out — until they're at shoulder level and parallel to the floor. Return to the starting position, keeping your back straight and your body still through-out the motion.

This exercise, like the dumbbell front lateral that follows, is as much a toning exercise as a strength exercise. I've known professional athletes, men and women in great shape, who don't use much more than 10, 12 or 15 pounds on the laterals. So don't go crazy with heavy weights.

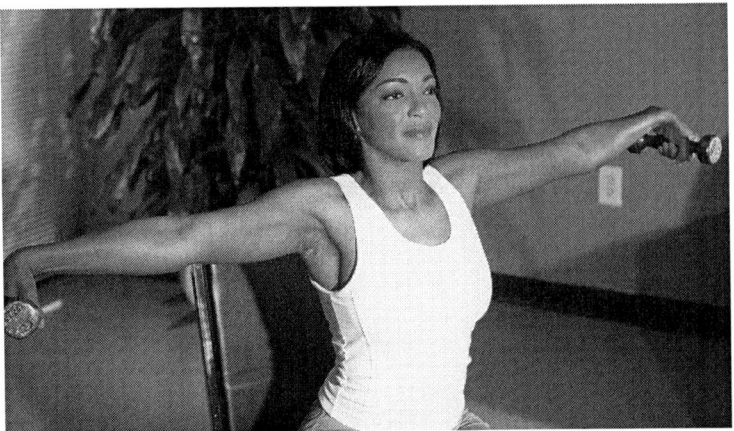

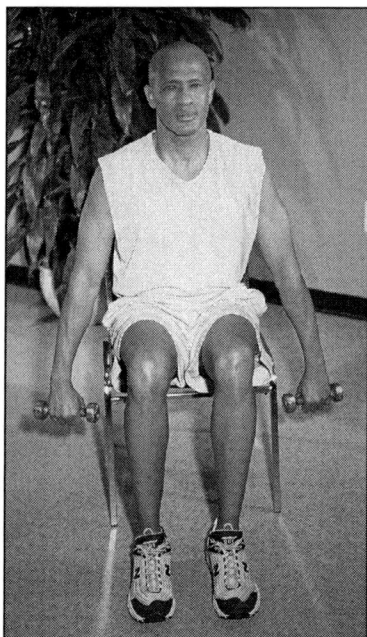

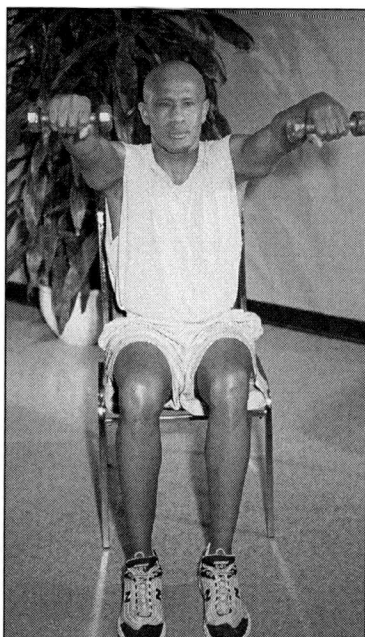

Dumbbell front laterals (shoulders)

Sit upright in the chair, back straight, legs slightly apart. Let your arms extend comfortably down at your side and grip the dumbbells with your palms facing behind you.

Keeping your wrist bent slightly and your arms straight raise the dumbbells fast in front of your body. When they are at or just below shoulder level, hold for just a second and then return slowly to the starting position.

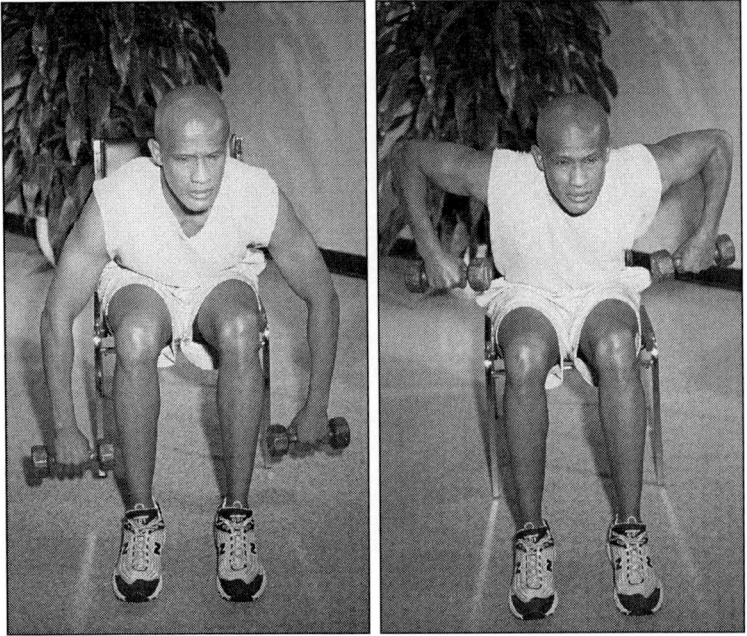

Forward grip bent over rows (back)

Sitting with your feet together, bend at the waist until your back is parallel to the floor. The arms should be extended fully down. Grip the dumbbells with your palms facing your body. Keeping your feet together, your back straight and your body still, slowly pull the weights up to the side of your torso as far you can, then slowly lower them until your arms are fully straight again.

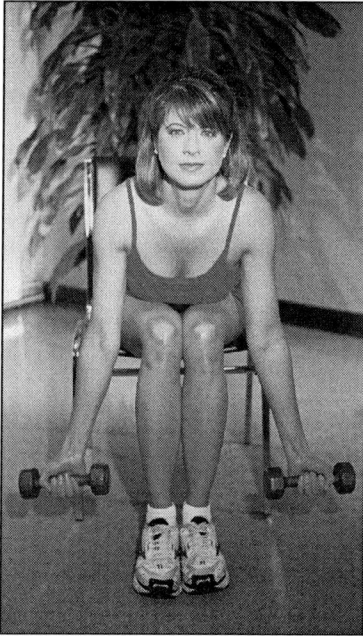

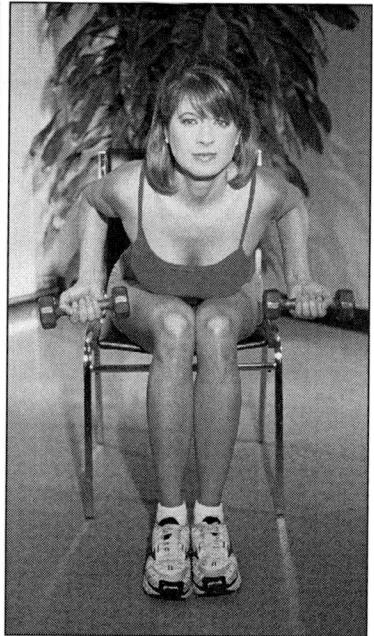

Reverse grip bent over rows (back)

This exercise is identical to the bent-over row with one exception: the grip. Your palms should be facing outward as if you were holding the dumbbell for a biceps grip. Other than that, there is no difference.

Raise the weights slowly up the side of your torso as far as you can, keeping your back straight and your body still. Return to the starting position with a smooth easy motion.

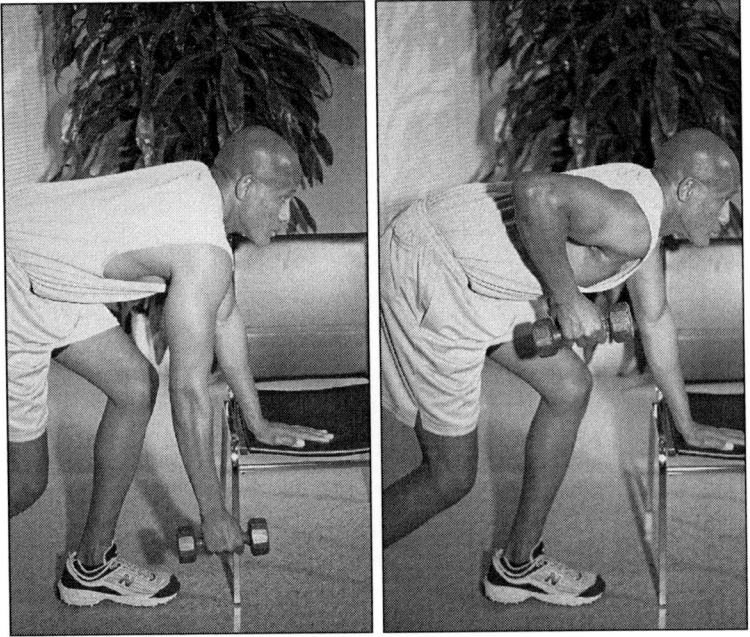

One arm row

Standing with feet together, step back far enough with one foot so that your back heel is off the ground and you are balanced on the ball of your back foot and your front leg. The forward leg should be slightly bent at the knee. Bend over so that your back is nearly parallel to the floor and with one arm support yourself with one hand on the seat of a chair. Grip the weight in your other hand with palm facing inward and arm full extended. Raise the weight up toward the waistline until the upper arm is parallel to the floor. Slowly return to starting position.

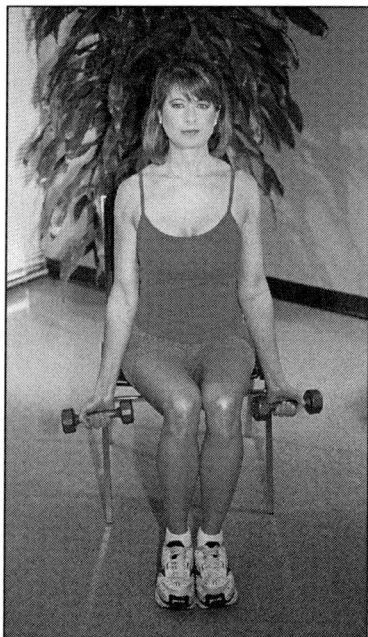

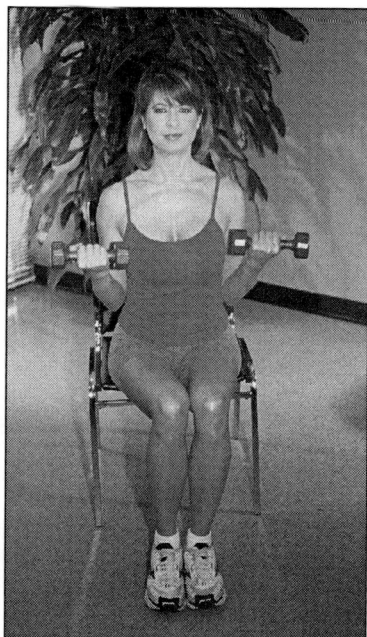

Dumbbell curl (biceps, forearms)

Sit upright in the chair with your back straight and your feet together. Let your arms hang down fully extended on both sides and hold the dumbbells with your palms facing forward. Curl your arms until your forearms touch your biceps, while keeping your elbows tucked to your side. Return your arms to the starting position using a steady, controlled motion throughout this exercise.

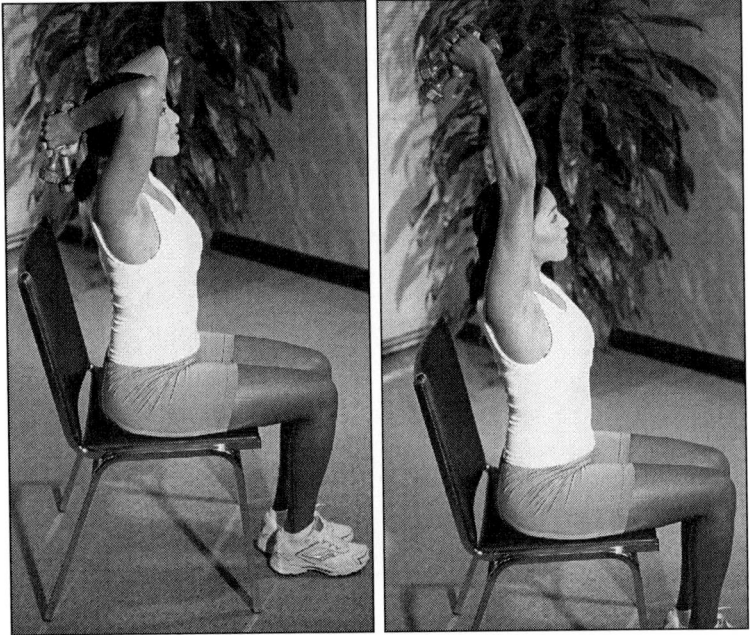

Two dumbbell overhead triceps extension

Holding a dumbbell in each hand, cross them over each other forming an "X" and grip them together with interlocked fingers. Seated upright in the chair with your back straight, legs and feet together and arms overhead with elbows bent so that the weights are behind your head, slowly raise the dumbbells straight up, gripping them with your palms facing in. Return to the starting position.

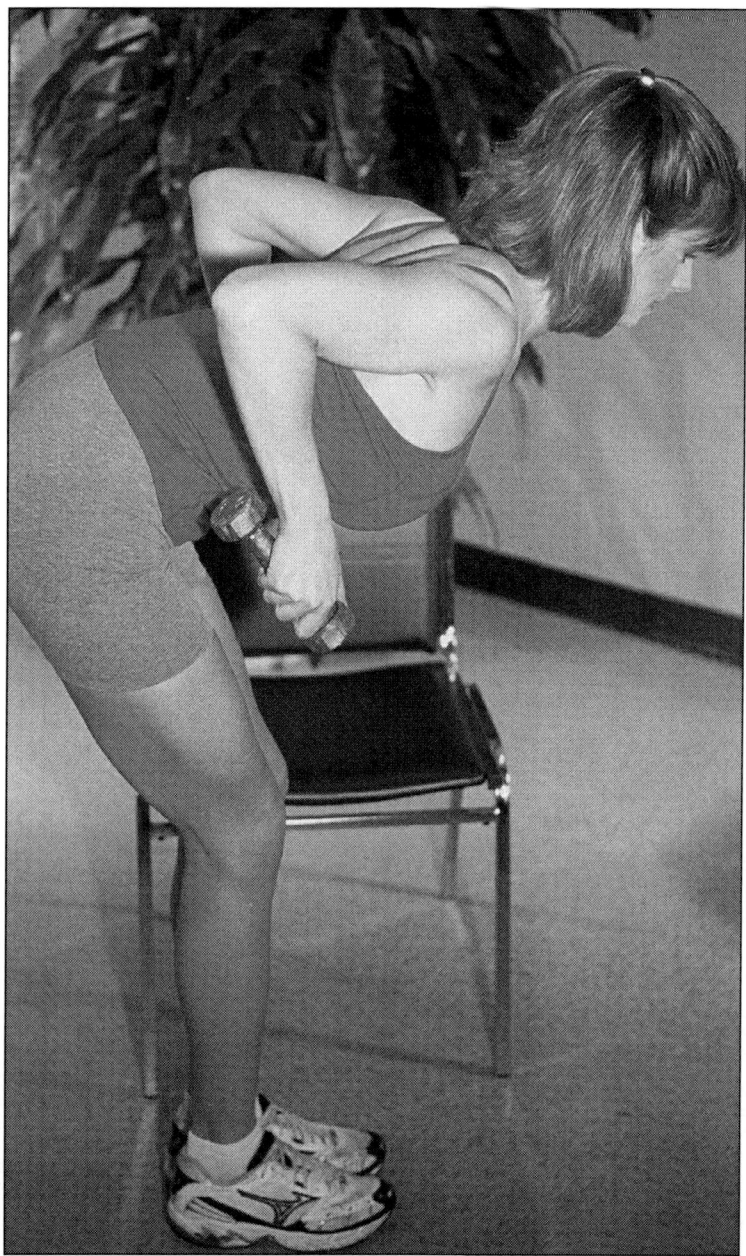

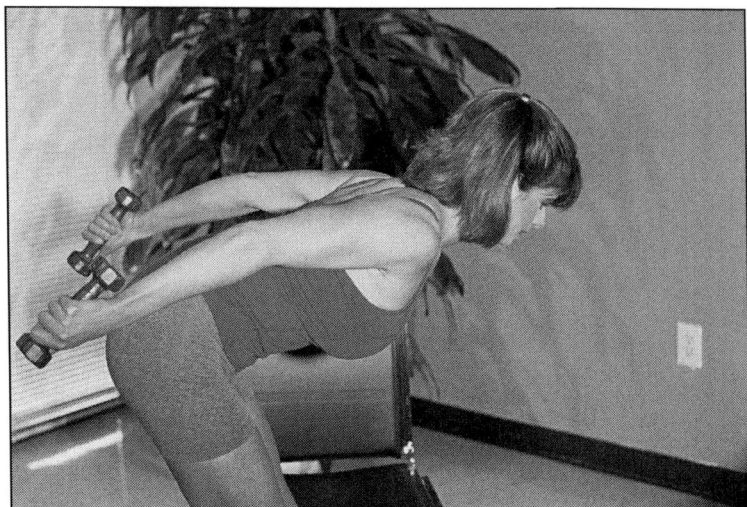

Two dumbbell triceps kickback

With your feet together and knees bent slightly, lean forward until your back is at a 45-degree angle to the floor. Bring your elbows up so that the weights are even with the torso and your upper arms are parallel to the floor. Grip the dumbbells with your palms facing in. Without moving your upper arm at all, extend your forearm back until it is straight. At the end of the extension, the dumbbell should be pointing down. Still keeping the upper arm motionless—pivoting only at the elbow—return the dumbbell to the starting position.

"Keep the lower body strong, and there's no stopping you."
– Ron Emmons

CHAPTER 5

Lower body

Let's face it.

When you think about getting in shape, you think about arms, chest and shoulders: maybe backs and abs. It's mostly those muscle groups whose tone, over the years, brings to mind the image of a strong, fit, well-muscled body.

So what's getting left out of that equation?

You guessed it. The lower body—specifically your legs and butt.

That's a mistake because those muscles are involved in just about any major body motion. Running. Jumping. Kicking. Even something as simple as getting up out of a chair or keeping your balance.

> "His legs are pillars of marble set on bases of pure gold. His appearance is like Lebanon, choice as its cedars."
> – Song of Solomon 5:15 (NIV)

For the most part, lower bodywork—at least in the Army—revolves around basic calisthenics, primarily lunges and squats. There's nothing wrong with that. It just doesn't give a complete workout to all the muscles you're going to be using throughout your life. I know a lot of people who think that if they run or use a treadmill, stationary bike or stair climber, they'll get all the lower bodywork they need. They'll get some, it's true. But they won't be strengthening every muscle: and that could result in a strength imbalance or, potentially, an injury.

Using dumbbells to perform variations on those standard exercises can help prevent problems. As I've said earlier, dumbbells force all your muscles to carry their own weight, so there's no cheating. Beyond that, they also give you the kind of resistance work that can maximize your strength.

> Dumbbells force all your muscles to carry their own weight, so there's no cheating.

Think about it. When you do a traditional squat, you're putting the body through the same degree of work when you lower it and return to the starting position. With dumbbells, though, you are asking the body to do more when you stand back up from the squat. That's resistance, and it not only puts some extra demands on the primary muscles you're working but also forces you to use some others that you otherwise wouldn't. Combined with the fact that resistance work produces quicker results, it's clear that dumbbells can boost your lower body strength significantly while avoiding many of the problems associated with standard exercises.

The bottom line is this: Your leg and butt muscles get you where you want to go whether it's across the street, around the track or over the training course. Keep them strong, and you'll be able to do it with less effort than you ever imagined. Better stated, there will be no stopping you.

The muscles

In working the lower body, we're talking about strengthening four basic muscles.

Quadriceps: The quads are on the front of your thighs and are primarily responsible for straightening the leg out. Because they play a big part in just about any motion, they're the real power in the lower body.

Hamstring: These are on the back of your thighs and they work opposite the quads. While your quads allow you to straighten the leg, the hamstrings let you bend it at the knee.

Calves: Located in the back of your lower leg, these muscles allow you to lift your heels off the ground when you run, walk or stand on your toes.

Glutes: We're talking mostly about the gluteus maximus here—your butt. It's the largest muscle south of your belly and is good for a lot more than you can imagine. It allows you to push your body up when you are running or jumping, straighten your legs out from the hips when you stand up after sitting and generally helps with flexibility and mobility.

The exercises

Before we get into the actual exercises, let me give you one word of warning. Because lower-body work does not include the kind of dumbbell lifting motions that were used for the upper body, people often want to use heavier weights right away. Forget about it. Too much weight can damage your muscles—regardless of how easy it seems—and put a serious strain on your back. Although I mentioned the safe starting weight levels earlier in the book, they bear repeating given this too-much-too-soon tendency:

Exercise	Weight Men	Weight Women
Dumbbell Squats	8 pounds	5 pounds
Angle Squats	8 pounds	5 pounds
Hack Squats	8 pounds	5 pounds
Stiff Leg Dead Lifts	8 pounds	5 pounds
Calf Raises	8 pounds	5 pounds

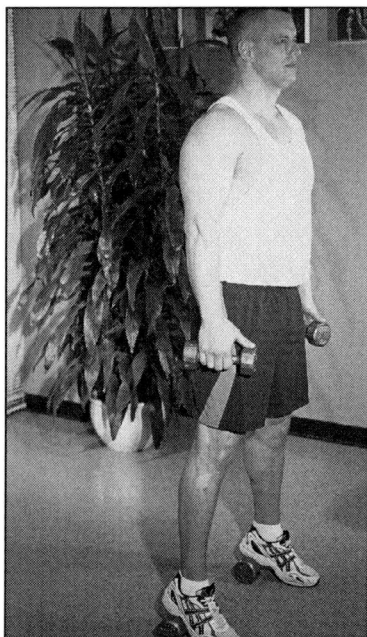

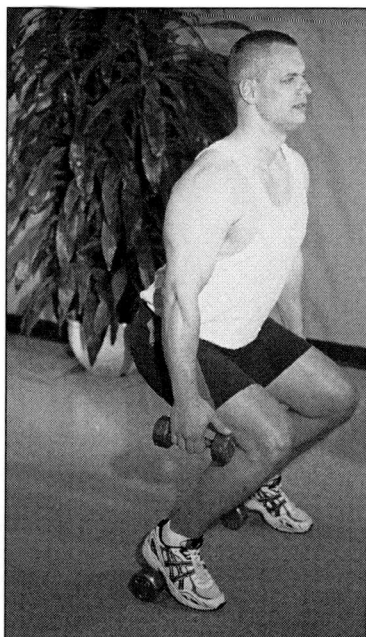

Dumbbell squats

Start with the dumbbells in your hand, palms facing in, and feet a little past shoulder-width apart. (For better arch support, you might want to consider standing with your heels on a 2-foot-long 2 x 4 or each foot on small hexagon shaped dumbbells). Keep your back as straight as possible, and don't lock your knees.

Slowly lower your body by bending both knees until you're at about a 90-degree angle with your butt parallel to the floor. You'll feel the quads start to burn a little. Briefly hold the squat and then slowly return to your starting position—keeping your back straight throughout and not locking the knees when you're finished.

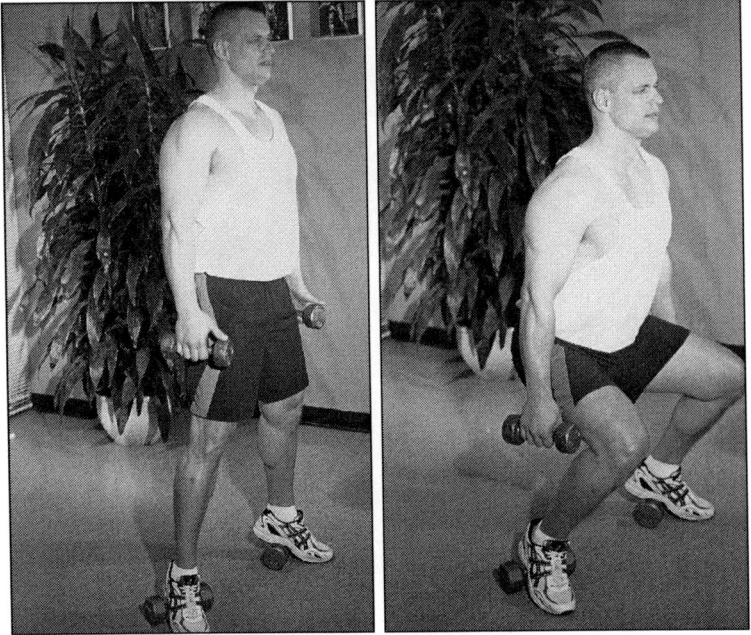

Angled leg squats

This exercise works the inner portion of the quad. Stand with your back straight and knees bent slightly. Hold the dumbbells in front of you, end to end, as close together as possible, with your palms facing in. Keep your feet shoulder-width apart but angle them outward at about a 45-degree angle. (Left foot pointed at 10 o'clock and the right foot pointed at 2 o'clock.)

Now, lower your body slowly to the point where the thighs are about parallel with the floor. Try to keep your back straight and don't let the dumbbells swing apart. Once you're in the squat, hold the position for a briefly before returning to the starting position. Be careful of one thing on this exercise, once your thighs are parallel to the floor-even if you feel you can go a little further- don't do it. When you get that low, you take some of the pressure off your quads, and you'll reduce the benefit of the exercise.

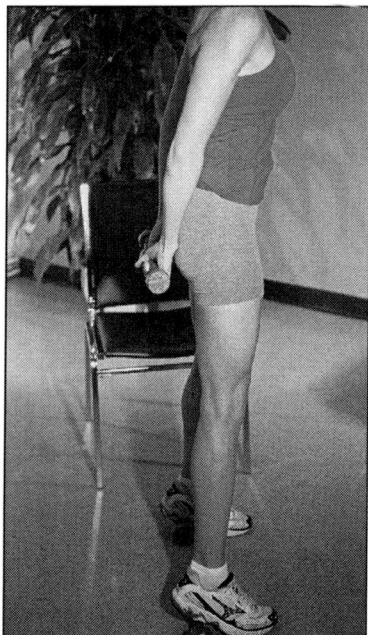

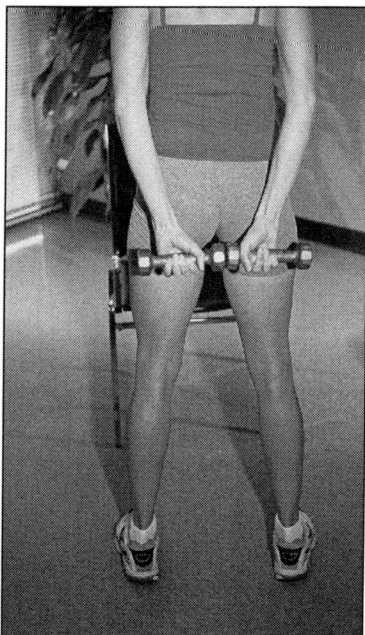

Dumbbell hack squat

This basically follows the same motion as the dumbbell squat with one difference: where you hold the dumbbells. Start with your back straight, knees bent slightly and feet shoulder-width apart. This time, however, keep the dumbbells behind you against the butt with palms facing away from the body.

Then ease down, nice and slowly, using the same form as in the dumbbell squats. Hold briefly and then return to the starting position, maintaining an easy, constant motion. The hack squat targets your quads, but it focuses on the lower part of the muscle that is commonly referred to as the teardrop.

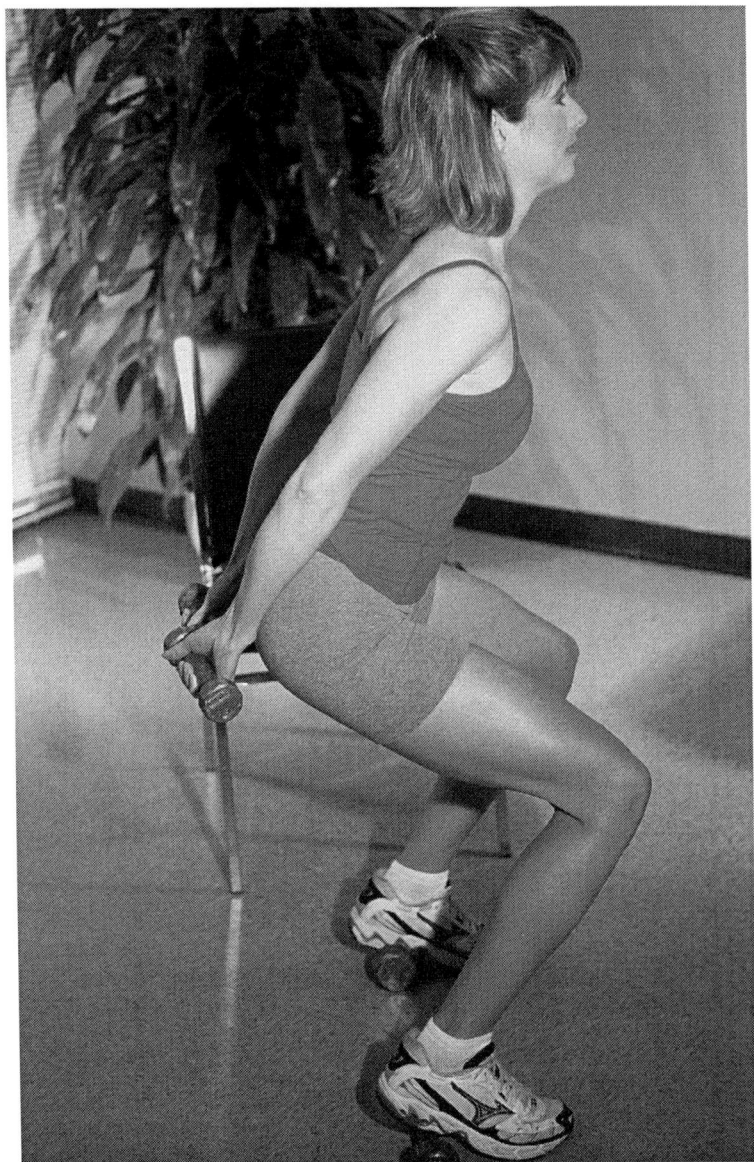

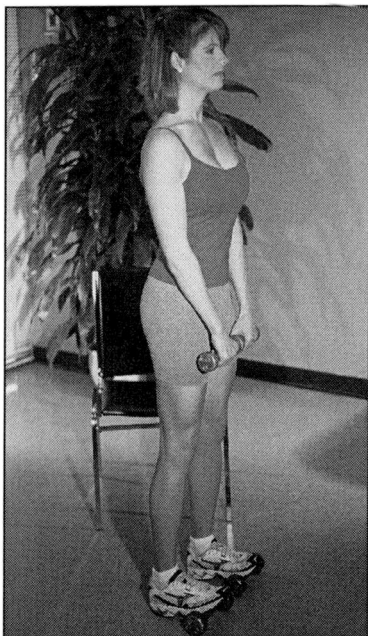

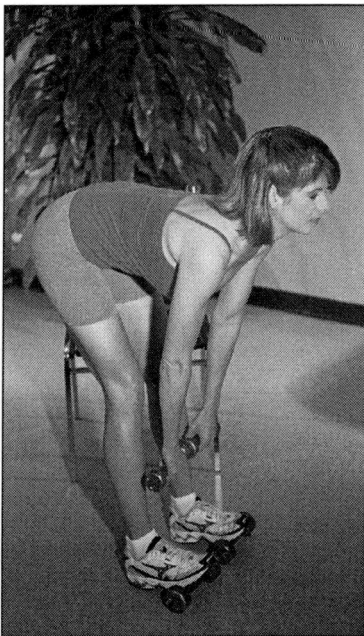

Stiff-legged dead lifts

Stand with your heels together and hold the dumbbells in front of you with palms facing in. Bending at the waist, keeping the legs stiff, slowly extend your upper body down to where it's parallel with the floor. As you return to the standing position, squeeze your buttocks together.

This exercise works the lower back and hamstrings, and the muscle contractions you make when rising strengthen the gluts.

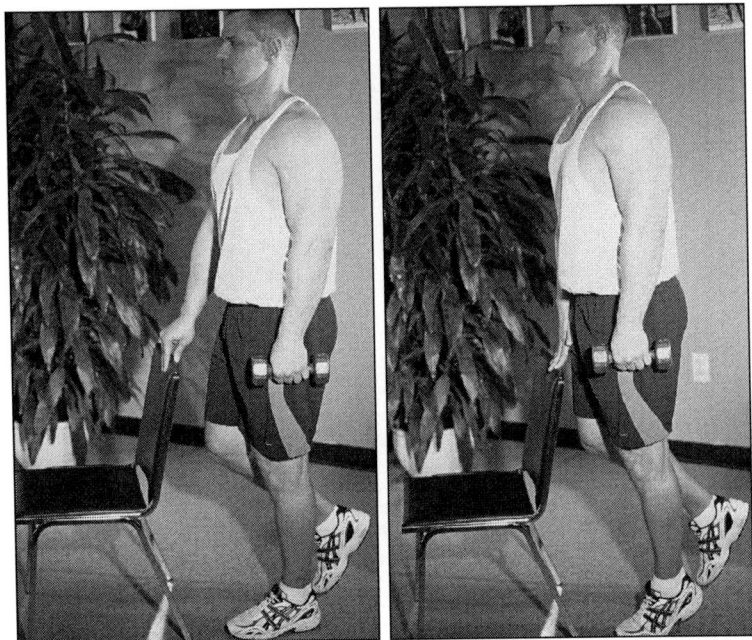

Calf raises

Standing with your head and back straight, grab something sturdy with your right hand—a bench is fine—and hold a dumbbell in your left. With your right leg out of the way, rise up on the toes of your left foot. Go as high as you can and maintain that position for a moment. Then, return slowly to your starting position while keeping your movements smooth, even and easy. Once you've completed the reps with one leg, switch to the other.

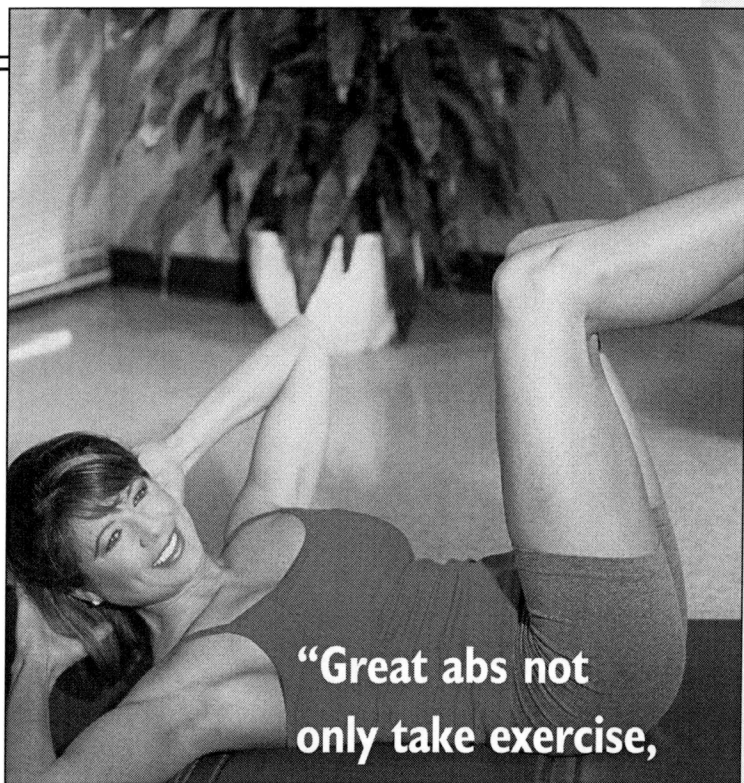

"Great abs not only take exercise, but proper diet as well."

– Ron Emmons

CHAPTER 6

Abdominals

You've seen them, just like I have.

Maybe it's a relative. Maybe it's a close friend. Maybe it's somebody in your neighborhood. They're carrying some extra pounds around the middle, or they're just too tight in all the wrong places, or their morning run seems more like a forced march. And you might think, sit-ups alone could give them the stomach and abs that they want.

> "What strength he has in his loins, what power in the muscles of his belly."
>
> – Job 40:16 (NIV)

Well, yes and no.

The truth is, the only real way to fight fat is with a proper diet and aerobic exercise. If you want to get rid of flab, you have to eat right and burn calories. End of discussion. Along those same lines, forget any talk you've heard about "spot-reducing". The idea that if you do a bunch of sit-ups, you can shrink your waist is a nice thought, and a lot of people have bought into it. But believe me: It's pure fiction. However, what you will get by doing a lot of sit-ups are strong abdominal muscles, and that's a good thing.

When we talk about the abs, we're basically talking about two muscle groups. The rectus abdominus, which are two thin strips of muscles run from the breastplate to the groin area. The others are the left and right obliques, which run diagonally on your sides and wrap around your middle from the front to the back. In terms of what they do, it's pretty simple. The rectus abdominus helps you bend forward, the obliques help you twist and bend from side to side. Basically, they connect your upper body to your hips and your lower body, and they support the torso and lower back.

> If you don't work the abs, you run the risk of either hurting yourself or reducing your ability to perform a whole range of activities.

You may be asking yourself, what's the sense of working my stomach muscles if it's not going to get rid of the baggage? It's a logical question, and here's the answer: If you don't work the abs, you run the risk of either hurting yourself or reducing your ability to perform a whole range of activities. That means when it comes time for a real gut check, you are not going to have everything it takes.

Every time you lift something, throw something, kick something or swing something, you are using your abs. When you bend over to pick something up, you use your abs. If you're playing touch football and shift direction, you use your abs. Think of all those body motions and how often you do them during a typical day. Now imagine not being able to do them, even the simplest one.

That's what can happen with weak abs, and that's why strengthening them make sense. No, it's not going to lighten that load around your stomach. But it will keep you on the go, make any kind of physical activity easier and help keep your back strong. Of course, it also doesn't hurt to know that when you blend killer ab workouts with a smart diet and aerobic exercises, you could get the kind of washboard stomach that most people would die for.

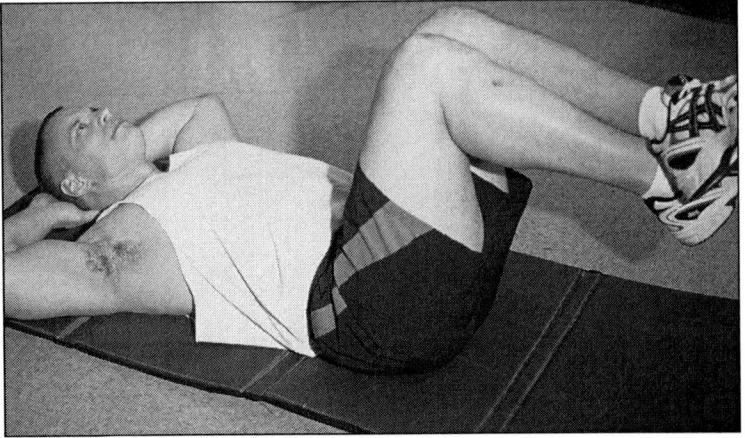

One final thing about exercising the abdominals. While it's always a good idea to give your other muscle groups a rest between workouts, you don't have to cut the abs any slack. **Work them every day and work them to exhaustion. You might want to consider focusing on your stomach muscles one day and your obliques the next.**

The exercises

I believe in crunches and standing bar twists. They work the abs and the obliques efficiently and effectively. They don't strain your back. And they give you a complete workout by attacking the muscles from every angle.

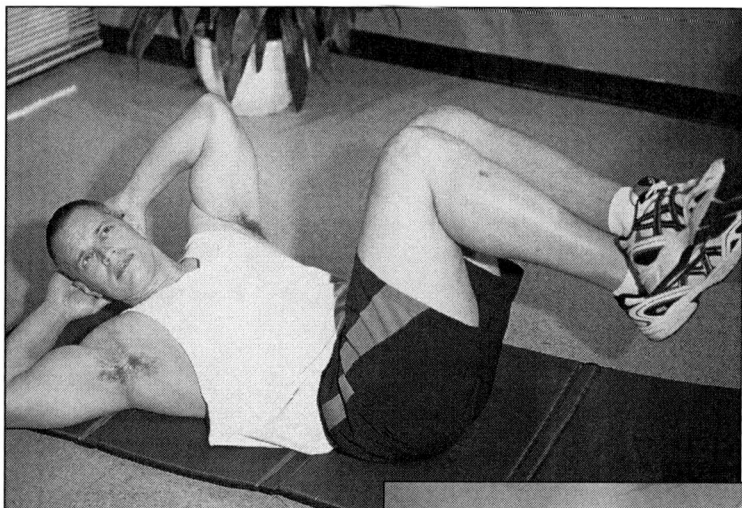

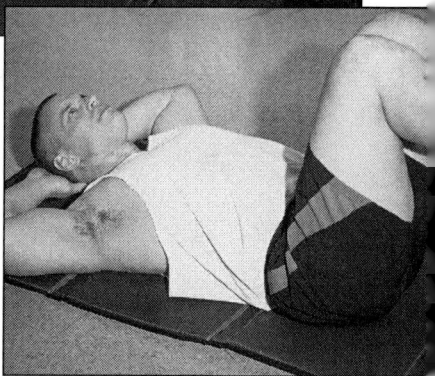

Crunches

Lie flat on the floor with knees above your hips and legs crossed at the ankles. Put your hands behind your head, fingers laced. Next, slowly raise your upper body only to the point that you feel your stomach squeeze and contract; this should bring your shoulder blades just off the floor. Be careful not to pull on your neck, because it can cause serious injury. Once you're up, rotate your torso towards the opposite knee and vice versa. When you've twisted towards both knees, slowly lower your upper torso to the starting position and repeat.

Do 15 reps in a slow, even motion without relaxing your muscles in between. Raising and lowering the upper body works the upper abdominal wall. Then, once you're up, the twist works the obliques. Crunches can also be done using a weight bench. Instead of bringing your knees to your chest and crossing your ankles, lie flat on the floor with your calves resting on the bench. Complete the exercise just like the standard crunch.

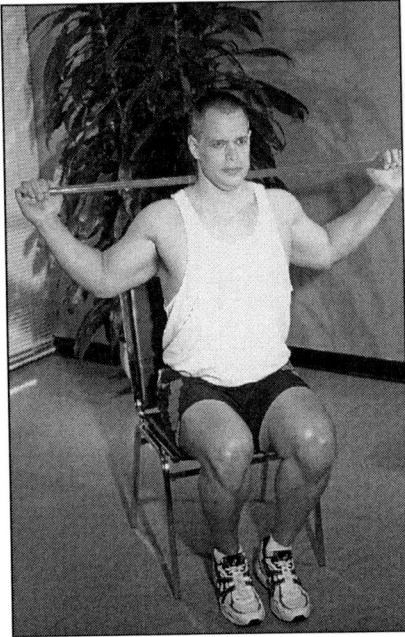

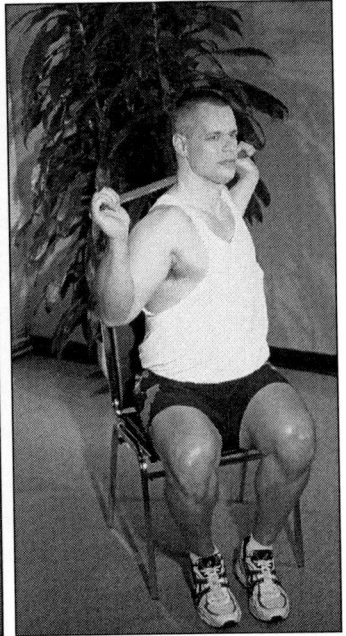

Seated bar twists

Sit upright with your back straight and your feet flat on the floor about shoulder-width apart. Rest a broomstick or something similar across the back of your shoulders so that it sits easily at the base of your neck. Keeping your head and hips still and your eyes forward, twist as far left as you can. Then in one complete motion without stopping, twist as far right as you can. Once again, keep your movements slow, smooth and as even as possible.

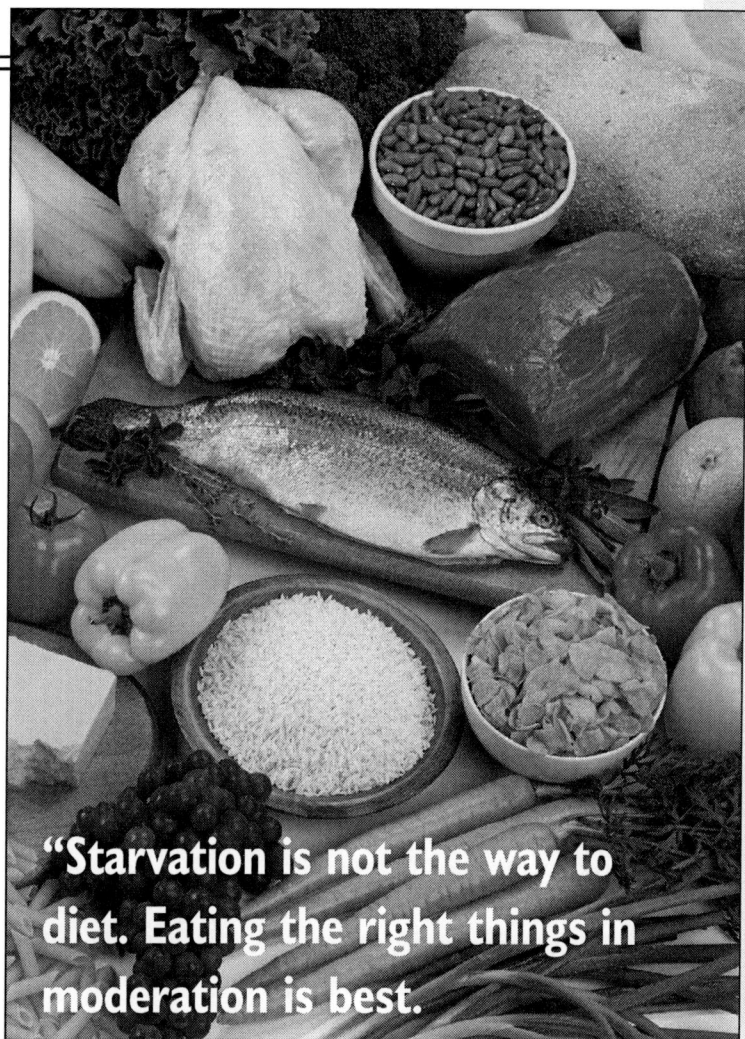

"Starvation is not the way to diet. Eating the right things in moderation is best.

Getting in shape is 75% about what you eat."– Ron Emmons

CHAPTER 7

Eating smart

You can't say enough about nutrition. Your progress in achieving personal goals is about 80 percent dependent on eating smart and eating tight. It's like putting gasoline in a car. If you put the wrong gas in, the car runs poorly. If you put the right gas in, it runs more efficiently. The body operates the same way. If you eat bad food, junk food or a lot of empty calories, your body is not going to perform to the max. So don't be fooled and think for a second that spending a lot of time on dumbbell training alone will give you what it takes to stay in shape. It won't. Good eating habits are going to make you or break you.

> "In the house of the wise are stores of choice food and oil, but a foolish man devous all he has."
>
> – Proverbs 21:20 (NIV)

I want to start this discussion by making a couple of points. The first has to do with calories. We've heard over and over that if you count calories or keep your calorie intake down, you'll lose weight. I hate to burst anybody's bubble, but as far as I'm concerned, calories are irrelevant.

What matters is how you're getting them—whether it's through foods that are high or low in protein, carbohydrates, fats or sodium—and how they're affected by things like your height, weight and metabolism. I can go on a 3,000-calorie-a-day nutritional regimen when I'm in weight training and still lose 20 pounds in eight weeks. In other words, don't get all wrapped up in this "Wow, I've taken in 2,000 calories today, I need to cut back a lot" kind of thinking. If they're healthy calories, they benefit you.

Next, let's get rid of another piece of conventional wisdom. You've heard all your life that three square meals a day will keep you fit, strong and healthy. Sorry, but that's just not the way it is. If you pack your daily intake into three square meals, your digestion will suffer. The body is not equipped to efficiently handle a lot of food at one sitting. Eating in volume makes you sleepy and tired and sluggish—which are three of the last places anyone wants to be.

Aim for five or six smaller meals a day: A light breakfast, lunch and dinner, with smart snacks mid-morning, mid-afternoon and in the evening. What this does is help you space out the amount of carbohydrates and protein that the body takes in, thus making digestion easier. Your body runs better, more efficiently and more smoothly.

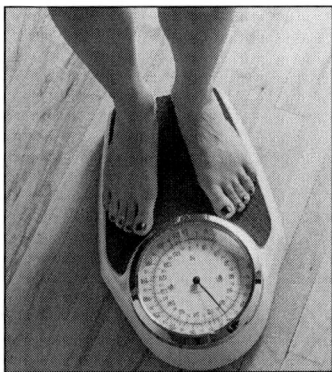

Nutrition for men and women

Men as well as women have to pay attention to four categories if they're going to eat smart: protein, carbohydrates, fats and sodium.

I'll skip the scientific definition of protein and tell you what you need to know: Protein is what our bodies need to build muscles and to repair them if they're injured. Most experts agree that protein ought to make up 10 to 15 percent of your diet; and, if you're really into working out, you probably need even more. Get less than that, and you won't bounce back quickly after exercising, increasing the risk of injury and taking longer to recover from an injury. Get too many, and you could wind up taking in fewer carbs so, when the body needs more energy, it goes for protein, which can cause muscle breakdowns.

So how much is enough? Let's take the example of a 200-pound man. Someone that size needs to take in between 1/2 and 1 gram of protein for every pound he weighs. That is 100 to 200 grams a day. Protein comes from a lot of sources.

But here's a list of some of the best:

• Jumbo egg whites: 8 grams per egg

• Can of white tuna in water: 35 grams

• Baked chicken, skinless (8.5 ounces): 29.2 grams

• White turkey, skinless (1 can): 34 grams

• Fish (4 ounces): 17 grams

Of course, there's always some debate about whether red meat's good for you or not. Personally, I don't have a problem with it-in moderation. Red meat is a good source of protein, provided you go for the extra-lean cuts. The operative phrase here is "extra-lean." I'm talking in the 4 to 7 percent range. So forget about a big slab of steak or a plate of thick, greasy pork chops. Sure, they'll give you protein. But they'll also give you a ton of fat and way too much sodium-two substances that will sabotage any effort to get in shape and stay in shape. **So here's the bottom line: if you're going to eat meat—and there's nothing wrong with that—eat it in the form that's best for your body and your conditioning program. In other words, eat smart.**

When it comes to how much to take in, you have to be careful too. You can only digest 40 grams of protein at one time, and it takes the body two hours to process it. That argues for spreading your protein consumption out over two-to three-hour periods and further makes the case for eating five or six smaller, lighter meals daily.

Your main meals—breakfast, lunch and supper— should take up about 75 percent of your daily protein consumption. Snacks account for the rest with large majority coming in your mid-morning and mid-afternoon mini-meals—a can of tuna or white turkey, for example. Or have a protein shake. Any flavor is fine, but try to get one that contains whey protein. That's the best kind for you. It breaks down easily so your body can process it efficiently. It's also the most nutritious protein source you can find—and it's a lot better for you than a bagel. When it comes to late-night snacks, though, don't load up on protein. Protein consumption in the evening should represent less than 1 percent of your total daily total.

Carbohydrates are stored in the body as a substance called glycogen, which is what muscles use for fuel. There are two kinds: simple and complex. Simple carbs come from fruits like strawberries, oranges and grapes. They're great for snacks being healthy and easy to eat. And because they're sweet—to say nothing of being high in Vitamin C—they'll keep you from reaching for the donuts, cookies, Twinkies and the other kinds of high-fat foods we all sometimes crave.

A lot of people think that because simple carbs give you a quick hit of energy, they will get you through a total workout. That's right and wrong. It's right, because the body processes the natural sugars faster and that does give you a rush. It's wrong because that rush only lasts about 10 minutes before you start to fade, so you're not going to get through much of a workout. The key is making sure you don't rely on them too much for your daily intake, but instead aim for a smart balance between simple and complex carbs.

> Aim for a smart balance between simple and complex carbohydrates.

Complex carbohydrates are a different animal altogether. They burn more slowly, giving you the energy necessary to get through a complete workout. You generally need at least as many if not more carbs than protein on a daily basis: 1 gram for every pound of body weight.

Some of the best carbohydrate sources are:

• Rice (20 grams for a half cup of cooked instant rice)

• Pasta (37 grams per one cup of cooked egg noodles)

• Baked potatoes (33 grams for one; keep the skin on, too, because it's got 4 or 5 grams of protein)

• Green vegetables (29 grams for a cup of canned peas, for example)

- Oatmeal (23 grams per cup)

- Bread (19 to 27 grams for two slices, depending on the brand)

One piece of advice: eat foods with complex carbs 20 to 30 minutes before working out. That will give you enough time to get the digestion process rolling and deliver the maximum strength you need.

Other advice about carbohydrates. **A good rule of thumb is that carbohydrates ought to make up about 50 percent of your daily diet.** But be careful. You want to make sure you're eating the right kind. Rice and potatoes are fine, but you still have to limit your intake of white starches because they can make your body retain water. Two final words on carbohydrates: First, never eat carbs by themselves. Mix in some protein. It will help you digest them better, so there won't be any carbs sticking around waiting to be turned into fat. Second, avoid taking in any carbs within two hours of going to bed because the food will just sit in your stomach undigested and end up stored as fat. If you insist upon eating carbs late at night, don't eat anything with more than 10 or 15 grams and don't plan on going to bed for a few hours either.

When you're talking about fat, it's a good news/bad news thing. The good news is that, if you eat smart, fat is no big deal. In fact, when you're work-ing out, you burn fat for energy. That means you're not cutting into your carbs, so they'll still be around to keep you from getting tired during the later stages of your daily exercise regimen. **The bad news is that too many fats can make you fat.** People talk about death and taxes being the only certainties in life. But I'll guarantee you that, if load up on high-fat foods, you're going to be looking at some serious spread around the middle.

The amount of fat you can take in depends a lot on how fast your metabolism is. I've seen young men and women who could pile on bread and potatoes and deserts, and still look like stick figures. I've seen those same people a few years later—when their metabolism has slowed but their eating habits haven't—and they're big as a tank. Taking metabolism into account, I recommend you consume between 10 and 15 percent of your body weight in fats. That's 20 to 30 grams a day for our 200-pound guy.

Since most fat comes from oils and animal products, it makes sense to avoid—or at least replace—those kinds of foods with

lower-fat substitutes. Remove the skin from your chicken and turkey. For example: a four-ounce piece of white meat chicken (roaster) without skin only has 5 grams of fat, while that same serving with skin has 15. Drink reduced fat or skim milk instead of whole milk. A tablespoon of apple butter doesn't have any fat at all; a tablespoon of butter has 12 grams. Heavy whipping cream has 22 fat grams in a quarter-cup serving; Cool Whip has 4. You get the point.

The final category of food men need to watch is sodium. Now, you can find no-fat foods, no-carb foods and no-protein foods. But if you're looking for no-sodium foods, good luck. While there are some exceptions—mostly foods with preservatives or additives—just about everything you eat has some sodium in it. A lot of that food has a lot of sodium. One teaspoon of salt has 2,400 milligrams.

A typical TV dinner can have more than 2,000 milligrams. Some canned vegetables run as high as 1,500 or 1,600. Tomato sauces push 1,100 or 1,200. The problem here is processing. In their natural state, most foods only contain maybe 100 or so milligrams of sodium. Start processing foods and the levels can shoot through the roof.

Sometimes you'll see people whose weight is roller-coasting all over the place—up and down and up again—and they have no idea why. They're eating low-fat foods, like they should but still can't seem to keep the pounds off. I'd bet that most of the their problem is that they are taking in too much sodium. The result is water retention, which works against all the other good things they're doing. It's an easy trap to fall into especially when you consider that 3,000 milligrams of sodium a day is too much (and remember, that's only slightly more than you get from a teaspoon of salt). **A good daily target is 1,200, which will keep the potential for water retention to a minimum.** So if you like popcorn or pretzels, get the unsalted kind. Eat a lot of vegetables. Cold cereals are good and so are crackers like Melba toast. Need a sweet fix? Have a Popsicle, raisins, apples or peaches. The rule is simple: Don't eat high-sodium foods. Period.

While we're on the subject of consumables, **I want to say something about water. Drink It.** Lots of It. Six to eight glasses a day. At the very least, it'll fill you up, and help kill off those nagging urges to snack or eat too much at mealtime. It will also keep you strong, too. It's no secret that you can lose a lot of water in the form of sweat during a good, tough work out. Runners can drop two quarts in an hour. The experts say that losing 2 percent of your body weight in water can cut back your endurance by 10 percent. So if you're not getting enough H2O, you're not performing to the max.

Especially for women

Although there are a lot of parallels between optimal nutrition for men and women, there are some important differences too. Much of it has to do with the nature of the body.

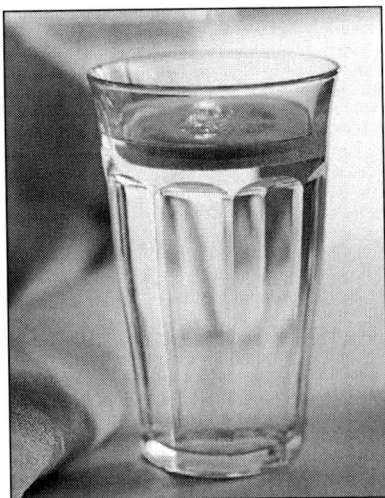

For example, women as a rule tend to have more body fat than men and they carry it in the hip area and upper portion of the back. This causes the metabolism to slow down, which in turn makes it tougher to get rid of excess weight. So women need to be especially conscious of fat intake and keep an eye on how much—and what kind—of carbohydrates they're getting.

In terms of protein, the rules for women are about the same as those for men: Take in 1/2 to 1 gram per pound of body weight. Get your protein in little meals every couple of hours throughout the day, not in three mega-doses during your three square meals.

Women especially need to be careful when consuming carbohydrates. Their bodies are carb-sensitive. So unlike men—who can take in a gram per pound of body weight and not worry too much about it—women should only take in 80 to 100 grams daily, max; any more and undigested carbs are going to pile up and turn into fat.

80 to 100 grams is a pretty good spread, so here's what I suggest: pick an amount in the 80 to 100 gram range, maybe 90 grams, stick to it for two or three weeks and see what happens. If you're getting the right amount of protein, you ought to be reducing body fat and, as a result, creating lean muscle. If you don't see or feel any change during that time—or you're gaining weight—drop your intake to 80 grams a day.

One simple way for women to cut carbs is to quit eating bread, at least until you have your body where you want it to be. Once you're in shape and your metabolism rate is fast enough to burn off fat, it's okay to eat a slice here or there. But select whole wheat.

Women should also take in slightly less fat and sodium than men. For fats, a good rule of thumb is 10 per cent of body weight. So, if you weigh 120 pounds, aim for 12 grams daily. And your target for sodium is 900 to 1,000 grams a day. If you can stay in that range—and keep the proper intake of protein, carbs and fats—you shouldn't have to worry about water retention or other problems associated with sodium.

Eating right

I have a simple formula for good nutrition:

Don't eat bad stuff and you will feel better. You will get the extra weight off and keep it off. You will get in shape faster and it will be easier to stay in shape and keep your body performing to the max. I'm not just talking about when you start your exercise regimen. I'm talking about all the time. There's no room for hit-and-miss approaches when it comes to physical training and proper nutrition.

To help you maintain proper eating habits, **keep a good diary, journal or eating chart.** Write down everything you eat, every time you eat it— main meals, snacks, all of it—for 30 days. It doesn't have to be fancy or perfect English. Create a record of food intake so you can see why you are gaining or losing weight. (If you want to take it a step further, make an eight-week chart that tracks both your food intake and your exercise regimen. That way you'll be able to see the direct relationship among good eating, exercising and body weight.)

It is worth emphasizing again that **weight changes depend on the amount of protein, carbs, fats and sodium you take in.** If you've lost too much weight or are losing more than you wanted, check out your diary. You're probably not getting enough fats. So put more in. But be smart about it. Don't load up on potato chips or a bag of Oreos. Get your fats from protein, not carbs. For example, you could add a four-ounce hamburger patty (not extra lean ground beef, but just basic ground round, something that will give you 10 or 15 grams of fat) to what you eat, and you'll start to see some results. That will help you put weight on gradually, and build muscles that are lean and mean.

If you are not losing weight or are adding some pounds, a quick check of your journal will probably show too many carbs and not enough protein. If that's the case, simply cut the carbs, boost the protein and kiss the extra baggage goodbye. If it doesn't happen overnight, don't panic. Losing weight (and gaining it, if you have to) is a process, which you have to do gradually—no more than 1 to 2 pounds per week. The important thing is to watch what you eat and keep adjusting the mix of protein, carbs, fats and sodium until you get the results you're after.

Ten recommended cooking or food substitutes

1. Equal

2. Sweet 'n' Low

3. Any salt substitute

4. Mrs. Dash (sodium free)

5. PAM spray (sodium free)

6. 1% or skim milk

7. Vinegar (as a salad dressing)

8. Mustard

9. Fat-free butter

10. Fat-free mayonnaise or fat-free Miracle Whip

The Temple of Fitness menu

So what's on the menu for maximum performance? A good breakfast starts with scrambled egg whites or egg substitutes like Egg Beaters, which have been defatted. To give a comparison, one egg scrambled in milk has 95 calories and 7 grams of fat; an egg white has 15 calories and no fat; an egg substitute has 65 calories and 3 grams of fat. Add some oatmeal and a piece of fruit—a banana has no fat and 26 carbs, an orange has no fat and 16 carbs. Top it off with 8 ounces of water and you're ready to face the day.

For lunch, enjoy a piece of baked chicken (without the skin) or fish, a green vegetable like broccoli and either a baked potato or sweet potato, with or without the skin. This will run you about 460 calories, 9 grams of fat, 60 grams of carbs, 140 milligrams of sodium and 40 grams of protein—max. Of course, you could have a Big Mac and small fries instead, and everything that comes with it: 870 calories, 41 grams of fat, 71 grams of carbohydrates, 1,105 milligrams of sodium and 20 grams of protein.

Dinner looks about the same as lunch, except for the meat. If you had chicken earlier in the day, have fish at night and vice versa. (The fact is, there are really only about four or five meats that are really good for you: turkey, tuna, baked fish, baked chicken and lean ground beef.) Try a different green vegetable, such as green beans—but not bathed in butter—and brown rice or another potato. Salads are fine too; lettuce is low-cal, no-fat and a great source of potassium, and a single large carrot will give you more than enough Vitamin A for the entire day. Just don't let a bad salad dressing drown out all the good. A single tablespoon of Italian dressing has 85 calories and 9 grams of fat, and blue cheese has tons of sodium. Instead, use a smart substitute like vinegar or a low-fat or low-oil substitute. If you want to turn the salad into a main course, that's fine. Skip the ham, cheese and crumbled-up bacon and add strips of baked chicken or boiled egg whites instead.

Snack times come mid-morning, mid-afternoon and, if you want, at night. For the first two, have a can of white tuna—packed in water, not oil—or white turkey; or, if you'd rather, a protein shake. A lot of people don't want to eat anything later in the evening, and that's okay. But if you do—and there's nothing wrong with it, provided you're not carbing out or eating fat heavy junk foods—consider something like rice cakes. They come in all kinds of flavors, are low in calories and carbohydrates (12 grams per half ounce), and have no sodium.

Ten recommended snack foods

1. Healthy Choice fat free snacks

2. Fat free cheese

3. Fat free chocolate

4. Reduced fat peanut butter

5. Unsalted almonds

6. Fat free flavored yogurt

7. Flavored protein shake

8. Fat free/low sodium chips

9. Sugar-free soda

10. Low sodium beverages

In the end, eating right is like doing anything right. You have to stick with it, be disciplined, see what works and what doesn't and be smart. I'll be the first to tell you it isn't always easy. But doing what's best rarely is.

Temple of Fitness eating plan

Breakfast

- 2-3 scrambled egg whites with 1 yolk
- 2-3 slices turkey bacon
- Small serving of grits or oatmeal with honey
- Piece of fruit (optional)
- Glass of water or orange juice

Snack

- 16 oz. protein shake or protein bar (20-40 grams of protein)

Lunch

- 4-6 oz. baked chicken or baked fish
- Small serving of your favorite green vegetable
- Small baked potato or small serving of rice
- Green salad with a vinaigrette dressing
- Glass of water or iced tea

Snack

- Small can of tuna or turkey

Dinner

- Same as lunch

Snack

- Plain or flavored rice cakes

(Note: Most figures related to calories, carbs, fats and protein come from Patricia Hausman's At-A-Glance Nutrition Counter, published in 1984 by Ballantine Books.)

Temple of Fitness eating plan for diabetics

Breakfast

• 2 egg omelet with tomato, diced, 1/4 cup onions, chopped

• 1 slice bacon

• 1 orange

• 8 oz. 1% milk

• 1 cup coffee or tea (use 1% milk)

Lunch

• 6 oz. baked chicken breast

• 1/2 cup red cabbage

• 1/2 cup corn

• Small baked potato

• 1 slice whole wheat bread

• Unsweetened tea (Equal or Sweet 'n' Low)—8 oz.

Dinner

• 5 oz. fish

• 1/2 cup spinach

• 1 cup whole wheat macaroni

• Green leafy salad (with Low-fat Ranch dressing)

• 1 slice whole wheat bread

• Water or non-calorie Beverage

Snack

• Mango

• 1 cup non-fat fruited light yogurt

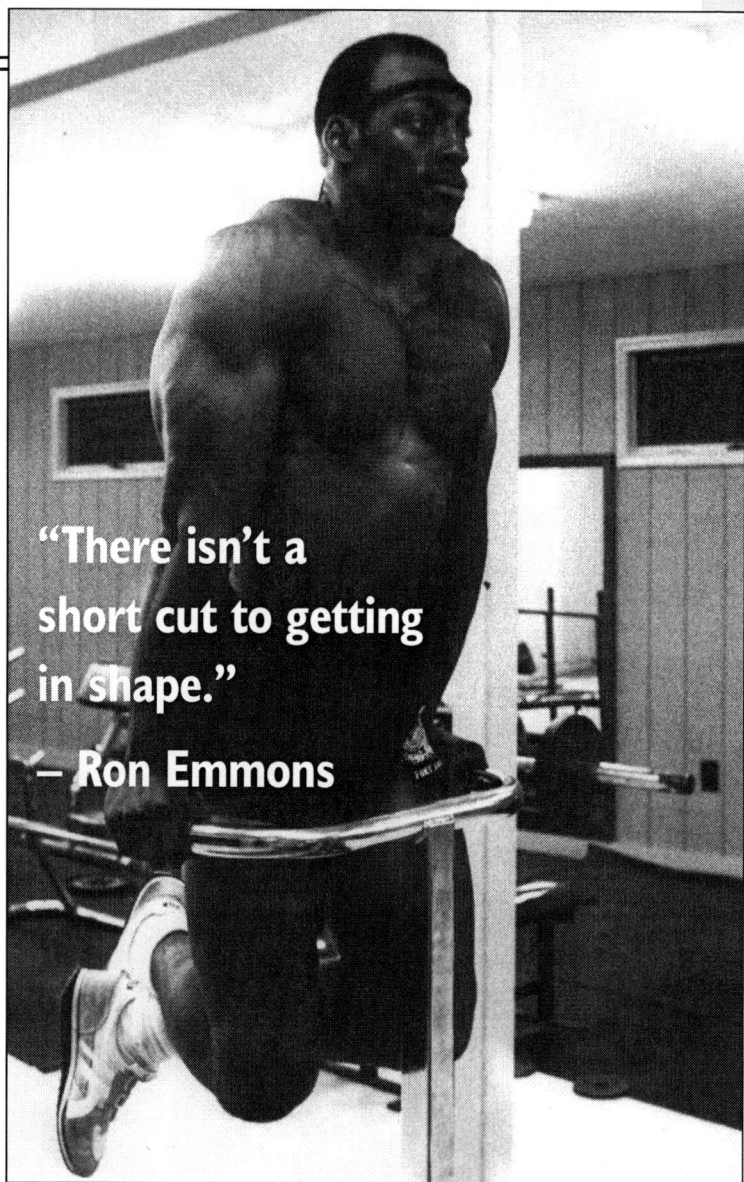

"There isn't a short cut to getting in shape."
— Ron Emmons

CHAPTER 8

Temple of Fitness

Workout

Staying in shape demands self-control, commitment, focus, persistence, character and discipline. There aren't any short cuts or an easy way out. Physical training produces both physical and mental toughness. Getting there isn't always easy, but the effort pays off big-time. You'll feel better. Above all you will have what it takes to meet the challenges of life.

"Therefore, since we are surrounded by such a great cloud of witnesses, let us throw off everything that hinders and the sin that so easily entangles, and let us run with perseverance the race marked out fur us."

– Hebrews 12:1 (NIV)

Temple of Fitness Workout for Men

EXERCISE	SETS	REPS	WEIGHT
Abdominals			
Crunches Regular	2	15	0
Seated Bar Twists	2	30 ea. side	0
Chest			
Seated Upright Chest Press	2	15	5
Seated Upright Chest Flye	2	15	3
Shoulders			
Seated Upright Shoulder Press	2	15	5
Seated Upright Side Laterals	2	15	3
Seated Upright Front Laterals	2	15	3
Back			
One arm Row	2	15	8
Bent-over Row (Forward Grip)	2	15	8
Bent-over Row (Reverse Grip)	2	15	8
Biceps			
Seated Upright Dumbbell Curls	2	15	8

EXERCISE	SETS	REPS	WEIGHT

Triceps

Two Dumbbell Overhead Triceps Extension	2	15	5
Two Dumbbell Triceps Kickback	2	15	3

Lower Body

Dumbbell Squats	2	15	8
Angled Leg Squats	2	15	8
Dumbbell Hack Squats	2	15	8
Stiff-Legged Deadlifts	2	15	8
Calf Raises	2	15	8

Temple of Fitness Workout for Women

EXERCISE	SETS	REPS	WEIGHT
Abdominals			
Crunches	2	15	0
Seated Bar Twists	2	30 ea. side	0
Chest			
Seated Upright Chest Press	2	15	3
Seated Upright Chest Flye	2	15	1
Shoulders			
Seated Upright Shoulder Press	2	15	3
Seated Upright Side Laterals	2	15	1
Seated Upright Front Laterals	2	15	1
Back			
One Arm Row	2	15	5
Bent-over Row (Forward Grip)	2	15	5
Bent-over Row (Reverse Grip)	2	15	5
Biceps			
Seated Upright Dumbbell Curls	2	15	5

EXERCISE	SETS	REPS	WEIGHT
Triceps			
Two Dumbbell Overhead Triceps Extensions	2	15	3
Two Dumbbell Triceps Kickbacks	2	15	3
Lower Body			
Dumbbell Squats	2	15	5
Angled Leg Squats	2	15	5
Dumbbell Hack Squats	2	15	5
Stiff-Legged Deadlifts	2	15	5
Calf-Raises	2	15	5

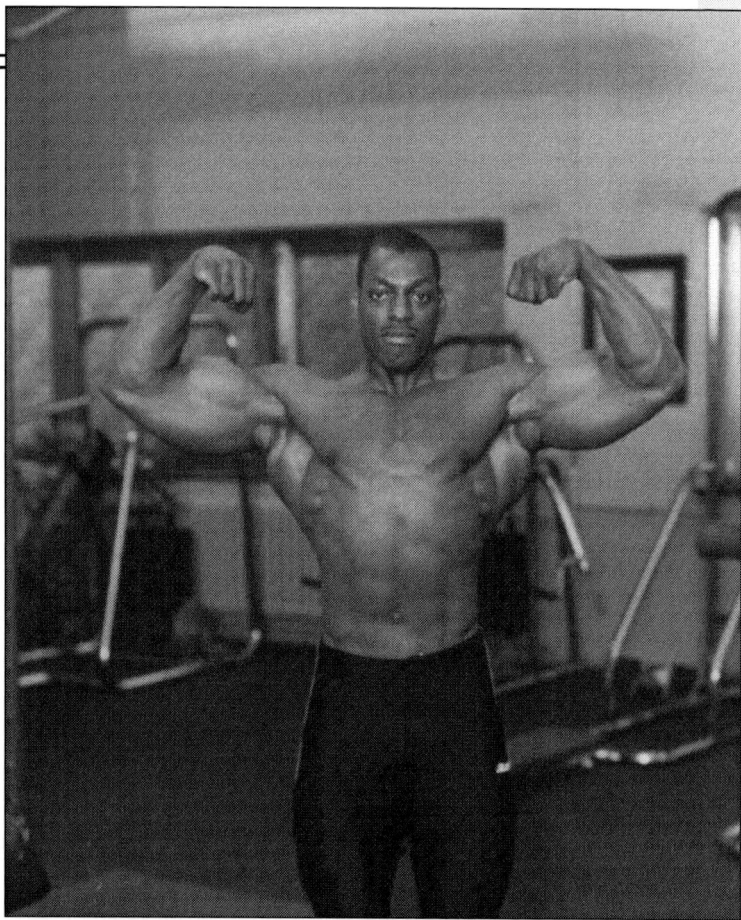

About

the author

Ron started his bodybuilding and fitness career in May, 1978, while stationed in Berlin, Germany, as a military policeman. In May, 1979 at age 19, he became the first and youngest American to win the 1979 Mr. Berlin Bodybuilding Competition. Ron went on to win 10 more bodybuilding titles worldwide, including the 1986 Natural Mr. USA and the 1988 Natural Mr. America before his career ended due to an injury in January, 1991. During his distinguished military career, he became one of sixteen military policeman chosen army-wide to be assigned to the Military Security Force, Office of the Joint Chiefs of Staff, the Pentagon, where he was responsible for the security of all the top military officers, as well as the Secretary of Defense. While stationed overseas Ron attended the University of Maryland and Central Texas College. In 1986 he taught "The Principles of Weight Training" for Central Texas College. Upon retiring from the U.S. Army in August, 1995, Ron began Ron Emmons Personal Training. He currently resides in Columbia, South Carolina with his wife and daughter where he works as a fitness consultant.

A lifetime steroid-free body builder, Ron has competed in many body building competitions.

Other major body building titles include:

• International Mr. Berlin 1979/1986

• Armed Forces Mr. Quantico 1985

• Mr. Washington D.C. 1985

• Natural Mr. USA 1986

• Natural Mr. America 1988

• 7th Place Natural Mr. Universe 1990

Photo Gallery

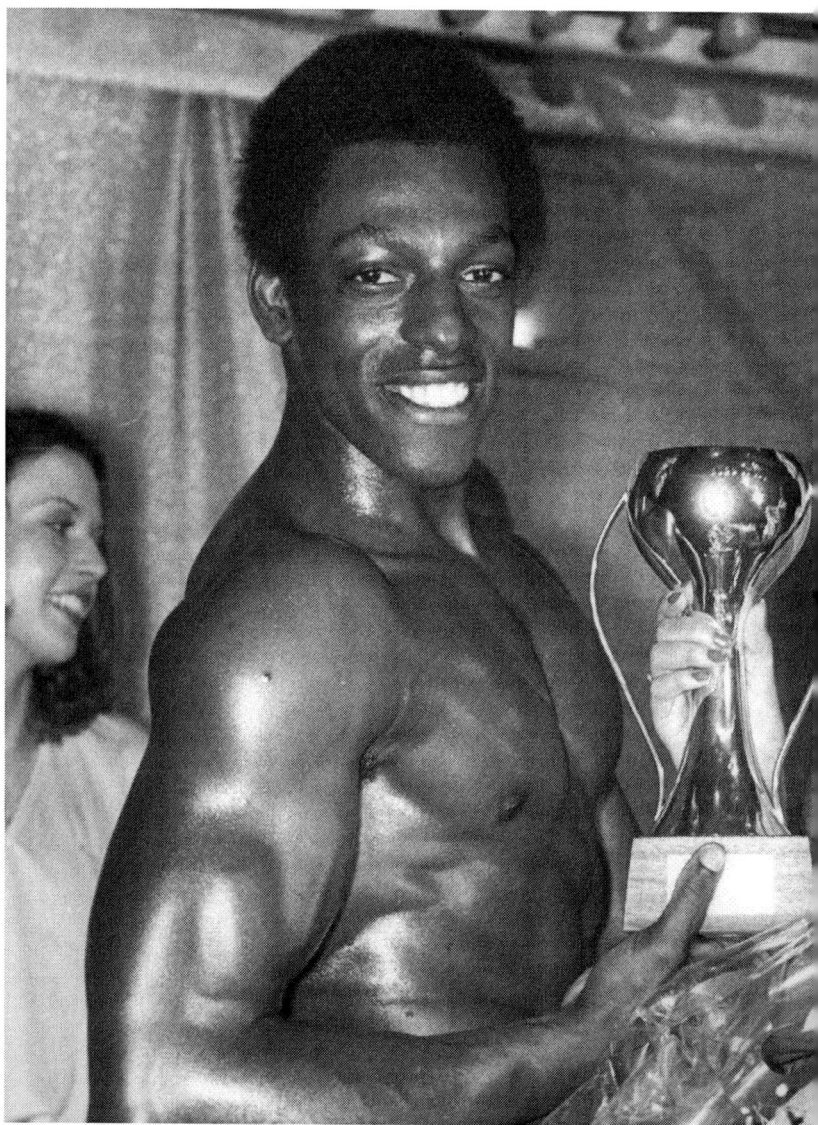

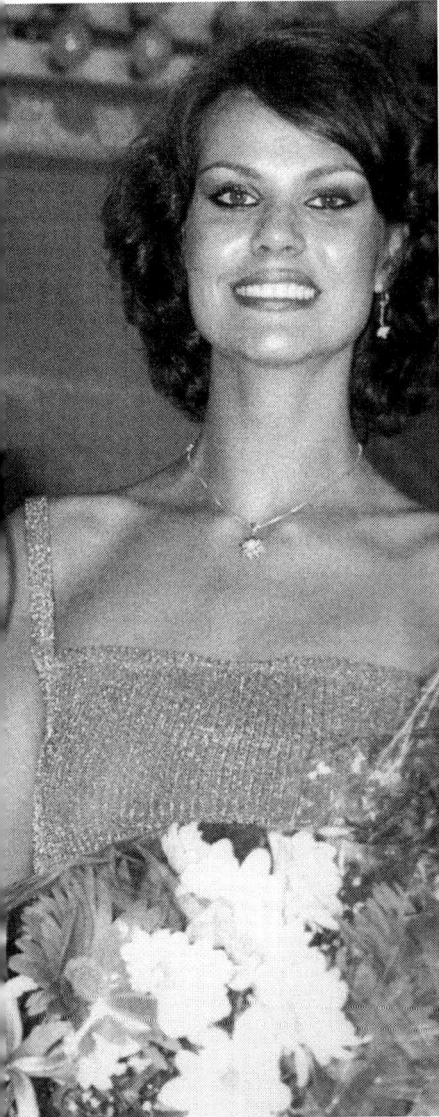

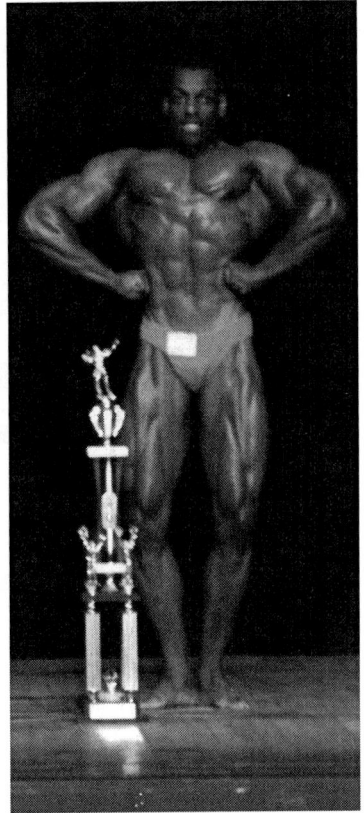

Left: Ron wins Mr. Berlin his first body building contest.

Above: Ron wins
Mr. Washington D.C. 1985.

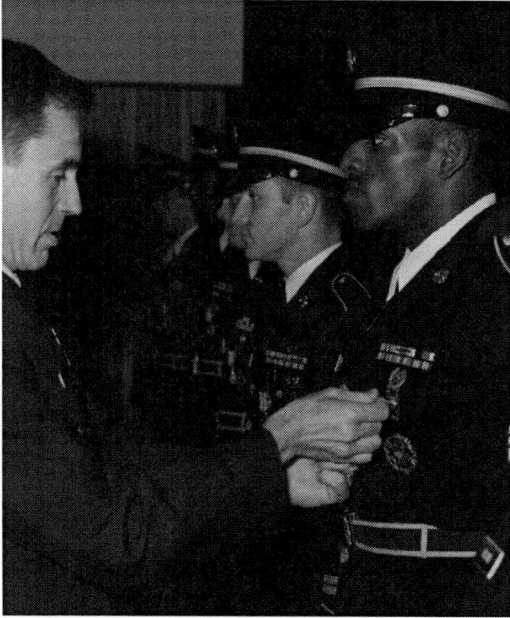

Left: Receiving
Commendation
Medal from
Pentagon General.

Below: Ron gets
promoted to Staff
Sergeant at the
Pentagon.

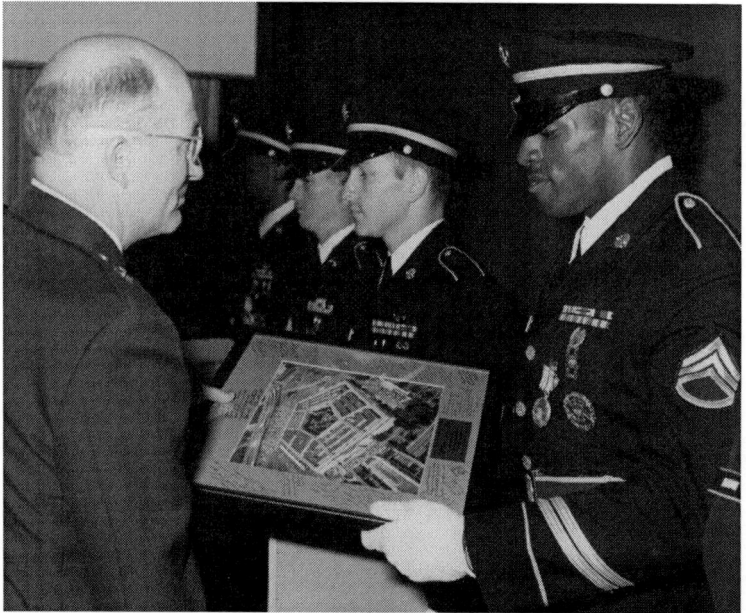

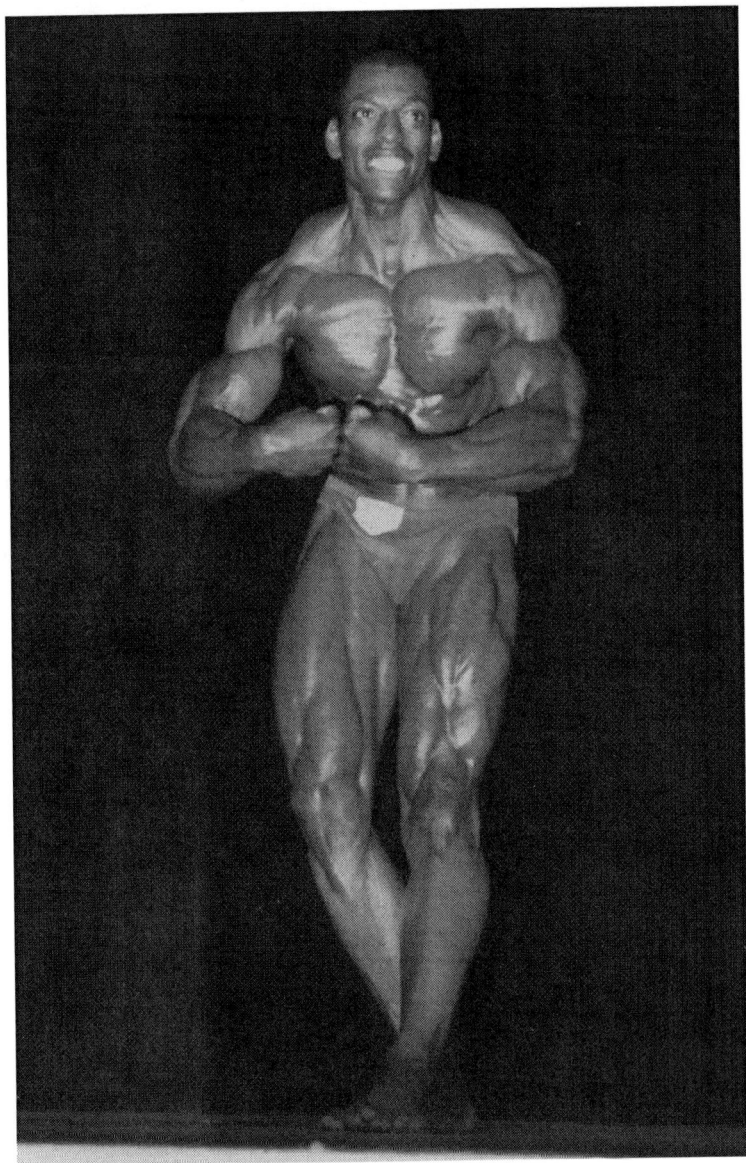

Ron performs at a body building competition.

TEMPLE OF FITNESS
Tracking Log

Name: _____

Starting date: _____

Height: _____ Beginning weight: _____

Body fat %: _____ Goal weight: _____

Week one:
Goals: _____

_____

_____ Ending weight: _____

Week two:
Goals: _____

_____

_____ Ending weight: _____

Week three:
Goals: _____

_____

_____ Ending weight: _____

Week four:
Goals: _____

_____

_____ Ending weight: _____

Week five:
Goals: _____

_____

_____ Ending weight: _____

Week six:
Goals: _____

_____

_____ Ending weight: _____

Week seven:
Goals: _____

_____

_____ Ending weight: _____

Week eight:
Goals: _____

_____

_____ Ending weight: _____

Week nine:
Goals: _____

_____

_____ Ending weight: _____

Week ten:
Goals: _____

_____

_____ Ending weight: _____

Daily journal

Week:_____

MON.	
TUES.	
WED.	
THURS.	
FRI.	
SAT.	
SUN.	

Make copies of this page so you can journal your daily progress. Use it as a daily record of training and diet. Be sure to record everything you eat, drink and do. Be honest, and don't judge yourself — this is about observing, not critiquing. You'll become more aware of how much effort you are putting into becoming a more healthy you.